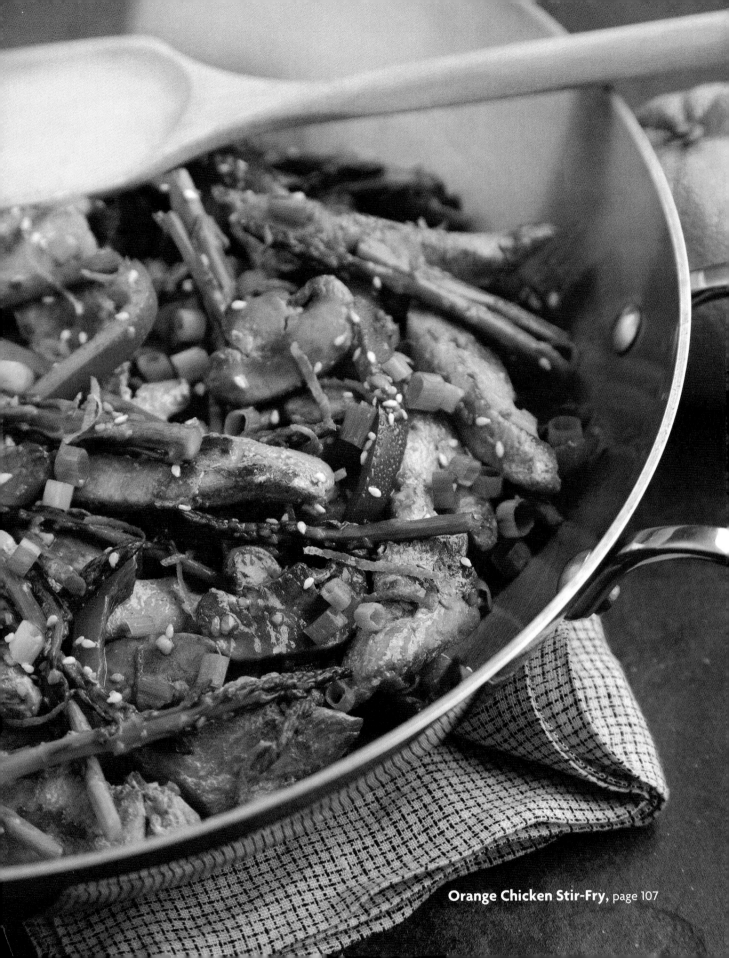

Orange Chicken Stir-Fry, page 107

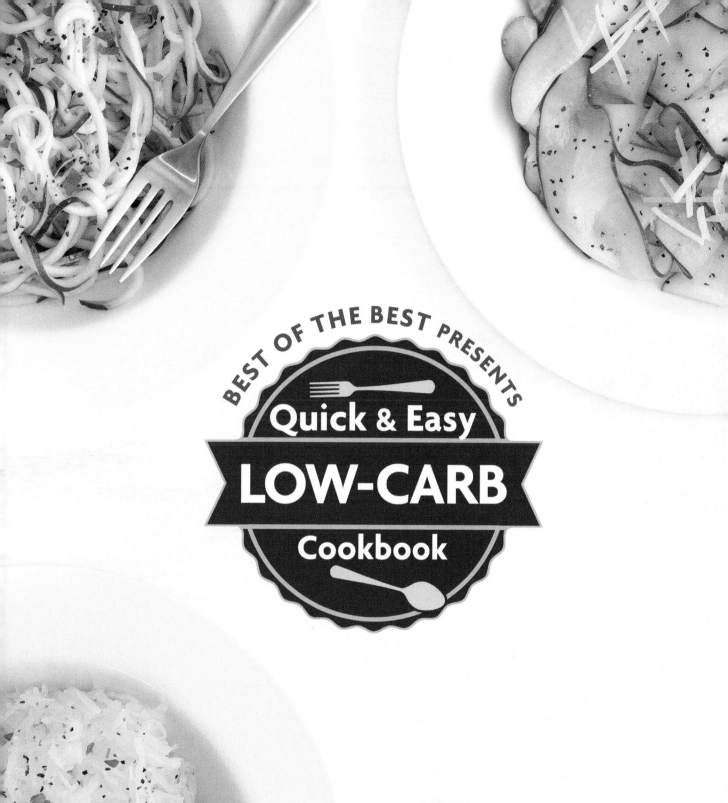

BEST OF THE BEST PRESENTS

Quick & Easy
LOW-CARB
Cookbook

GEORGE STELLA

WITH CHRISTIAN STELLA

QUAIL RIDGE PRESS
Preserving America's Food Heritage

Authors:
George Stella
with Christian Stella

Book Design and Food Photography by
Christian and Elise Stella

This book is not meant to dispense medical advice. Please consult your doctor before making any dramatic changes to the way you eat.

Nutritional analysis provided on each recipe is meant only as a reference and has been compiled to the best of our ability using nutritional analysis software. Due to differences in sizes, brands, and types of ingredients, your calculations may vary. Calories have been rounded to the nearest 5, and all other amounts were rounded to the nearest .5 of a gram.

Front cover: Coconut Cheesecake with Macadamia Nut Crust, page 219
Mozzarella Sticks, page 85 • Fork & Knife Meatballs, page 147

Back cover: Pepper Jack "Corn" Muffins, page 65
Chili-Rubbed Chicken Breasts, page 103

ISBN 978-1-938879-23-4
Printed in the United States of America
First edition

QUAIL RIDGE PRESS
P. O. Box 123 • Brandon, MS 39043 • 1-800-343-1583
info@quailridge.com • www.quailridge.com

TABLE OF CONTENTS

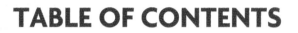

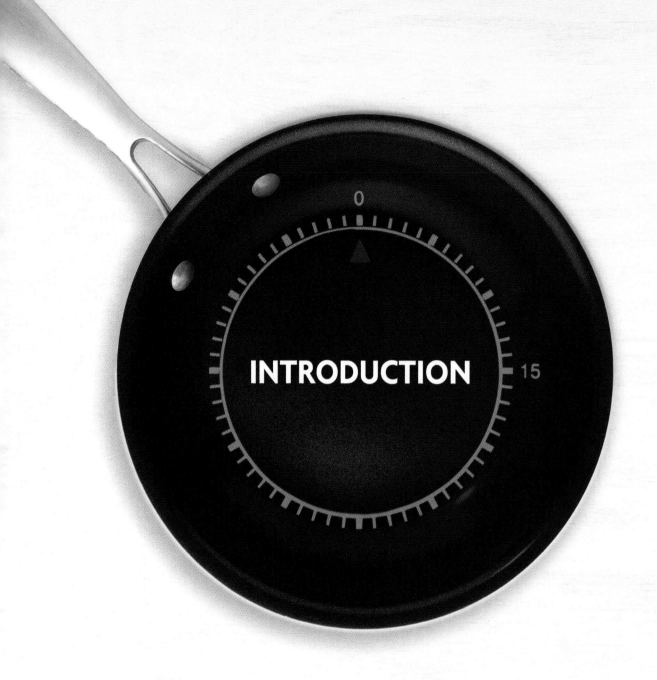

INTRODUCTION

MAKING A CHANGE

Making a resolution to change is *quick and easy*. It only takes a moment—a spark of inspiration—to decide that things can be different: that you don't have to continue down the same path or make the same choices. Things don't have to spiral out of control. You can resolve to make something better. Resolutions are so quick, so easy, that most people will make at least one every New Year…but we don't always stick to them.

It's been more than fifteen years since I made the resolution to live. I was 467 pounds with numerous health problems, including congestive heart failure, sleep apnea, and bout after bout of pneumonia.

When you're obese, you get used to doctors telling you that you're going to die…that this is the path that you're letting food take you down…a spiral that starts at the refrigerator and ends very grim. Doctors like to remind you of this. Confined to a wheelchair and sick with my third run of pneumonia in a little over a year, I finally believed the doctor. It no longer felt like just a nagging voice that was telling me how unhealthy I'd become. It truly felt like the truth. The doctor said I was going to die, and I finally believed him. My time was running out.

Somewhere along the line, my whole family decided to follow the example I had set for them. We had become a fat family, enabling each other in our bad eating. My wife Rachel—who had never struggled with her weight earlier in life—had reached 200 pounds. My two teenage sons were gaining more and more weight every year, with my youngest son Christian reaching 305 pounds at age 15. We all seemed to be resigned to the way things were going, and the size we had become.

We found out about low-carb eating at the perfect moment, when both my health

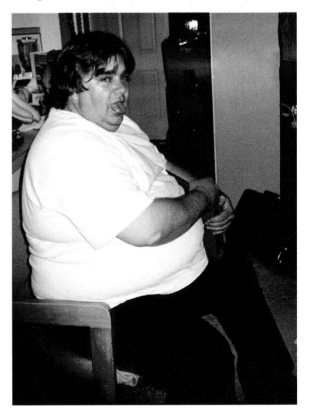

BEFORE...

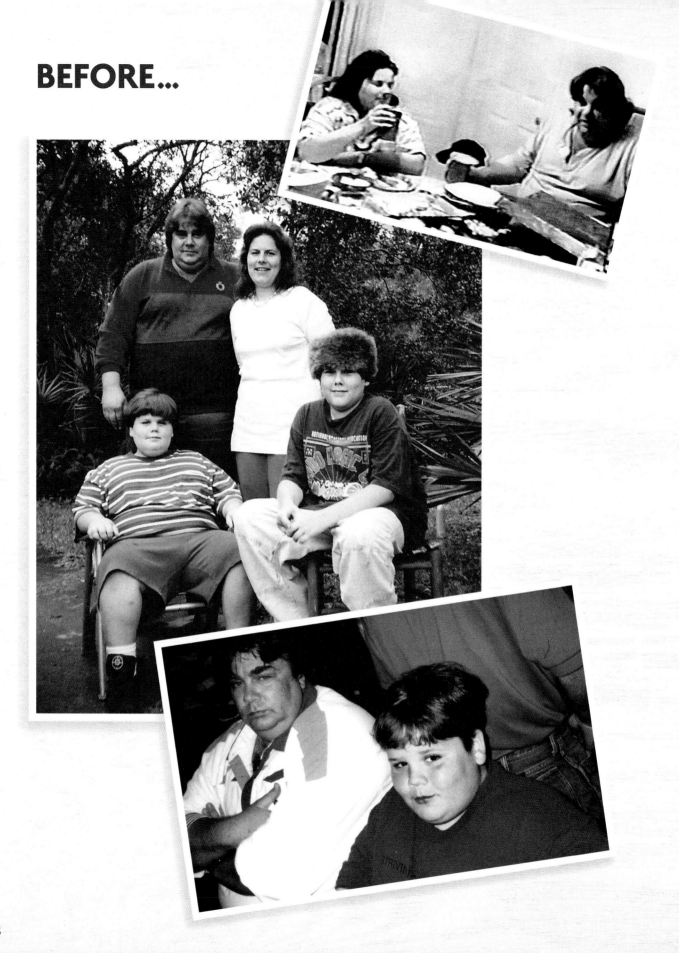

and morale were at rock bottom. It was that spark I needed to make a resolution I would follow through on. The concept of low-carb seemed too easy. The food seemed too good to be true. I wasn't sure it would work, but I was hopeful and willing to try anything. The fact that I could eat a steak on a "diet" seemed so foreign all those years ago, just as low-carb was first gaining awareness.

As a chef working in some of Florida's best restaurants, I had always loved to cook. The downside of being a chef is that you don't always want to come home and fire up the grill after 12 hours of cooking over a commercial grill. Once my health had deteriorated, I wasn't cooking at home *or* in a restaurant. I simply wasn't cooking at all. Low-carb gave me back my passion for cooking. It gave me the drive to cook for my family—and for myself—food of the quality I once cooked only for restaurant guests.

I soon learned that low-carb wasn't a "diet" at all. It was a lifestyle, and one I had no problem sticking to…a lifestyle my whole family adopted together…a lifestyle change with real results…results that start in the kitchen, cooking fresh and delicious meals made from *real* food. To eat well, you have to cook well. It doesn't have to be difficult. And it doesn't have to take all day.

True success can only come when you're enjoying the journey. Cooking should never feel like work, and eating should never be boring.

For us, success came quickly. My family lost over 560 pounds, and have kept it off for more than 12 years. Rachel and Anthony each dropped over 70 pounds. Christian lost more than half his body weight, going from 305 to under 150. I lost 265 pounds, got out of the wheelchair, and was finally back in restaurant kitchens—only this time I didn't do all the cooking in the workplace.

I wasn't just cooking at home; I was developing new dishes. I was reinventing comfort foods to fit into our low-carb lifestyle. My family never felt like we had to go without, and we kept perfecting our recipes every day of our weight loss.

It has been over a decade since my first cookbook of low-carb recipes was published, and we're still in the kitchen cooking. We're still living a low-carb lifestyle and loving every minute of it. We're still developing brand new recipes and perfecting old techniques. But we understand that not everyone has this kind of time to devote to cooking.

The recipes in this book are "Quick & Easy" but still made from fresh, naturally low-carb ingredients. They're everyday recipes that anyone can cook, no matter their skill level. They're the results of years of trial, error, and reinventing—simplified, but not to the point that they have no flavor. I've done my best to keep the shopping lists to a minimum, without skimping on the pantry ingredients and spices that make a dish shine. There are plenty of "5-ingredient" cookbooks out there, but I can't bring myself to leave out something as simple as pepper, just to fit an arbitrary number. I am a chef after all. And I truly love food.

These recipes are proof that things can be different. Pasta can be something better for you. A diet can be a "lifestyle." Resolutions can stick. Lives can change.

I'm living proof.

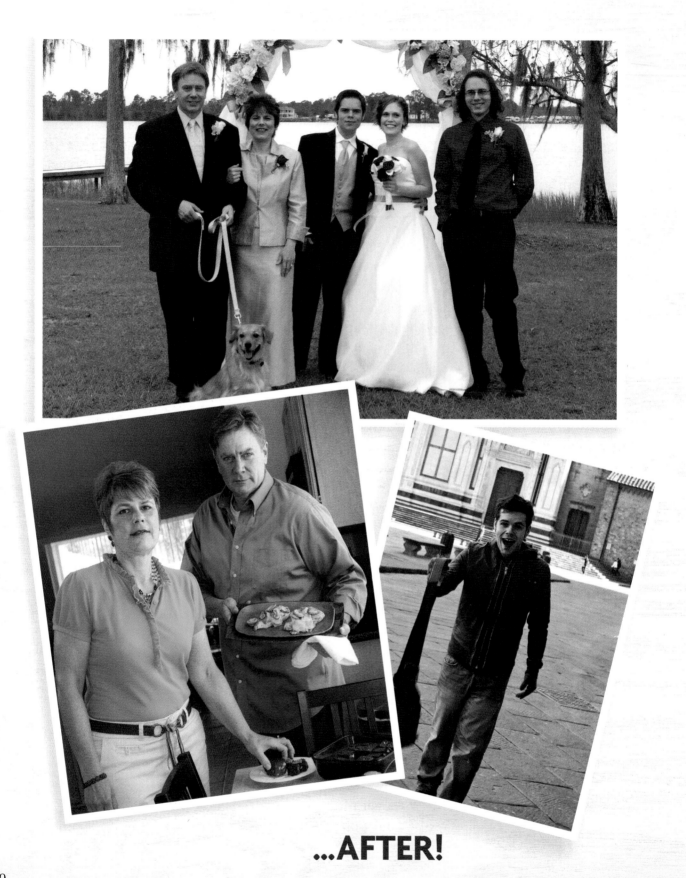

...AFTER!

HOW LOW-CARB WORKS

First and foremost, I am a chef, not a doctor, nutritionist, or scientist. My experiments are with ingredients, not test tubes. The good news is… This is a cookbook! You wouldn't want a doctor writing recipes (many have), but you should consult a doctor or nutritionist before making changes to the way you eat.

You should also understand that my explanation of how low-carb works is extremely simplified and based on my own experience of losing weight. The specifics of what is actually happening inside the body to lead to weight loss is beyond the scope of this cookbook, but something you may want to further research. I would highly suggest Dr. Atkins New Diet Revolution, as that is the book that we read before starting our own personal journeys. It's very long, very technical, but pretty much the go-to reference book on low-carb by the man who started it all, Robert Atkins.

Now, reading a 500+ page reference book isn't exactly "Quick & Easy," so here is my simplification of why and how low-carb works.

STORING FAT

The concept of eating low-carb is actually quite simple to explain. Our bodies are capable of converting either carbohydrates or fat into the energy needed to function; however, our bodies prefer carbohydrates when they are available. Eating a diet full of carbohydrates causes the body to burn only the carbs necessary to get through the day before then converting the remaining carbohydrates into fat, which is then stored—alongside the actual fat you eat—in the event there ever comes a time when excess fat is needed for survival. This is the reason that overeating leads to weight gain. When eating an abundance of carbohydrates alongside fat, we are similar to bears storing fat for hibernation in the winter.

BURNING FAT

Your body can also create energy from fat when it is not supplied with an ample amount of carbohydrates. By converting fat into energy, your body goes into a constant fat-burning state known as "ketosis." Not only do you burn the fat that you eat, you can also burn through your reserved fat. Most people find it hard to grasp why low-carb allows you to eat fattier foods. There's a simple explanation—your body burns it right off.

Entering the "ketosis" state is easily achieved; simply stop eating processed carbohydrates. If you are looking to lose weight, staying in a state of ketosis is important to success. Cheating on a low-carb lifestyle will take your body out of ketosis and stop burning fat.

For me, the best judge of whether my body was in ketosis, was whether I was losing weight from week to week (don't weigh yourself daily or you'll go crazy). That said, you can also purchase very inexpensive test strips at most pharmacies or superstores. They will be labeled as "ketone test strips,"

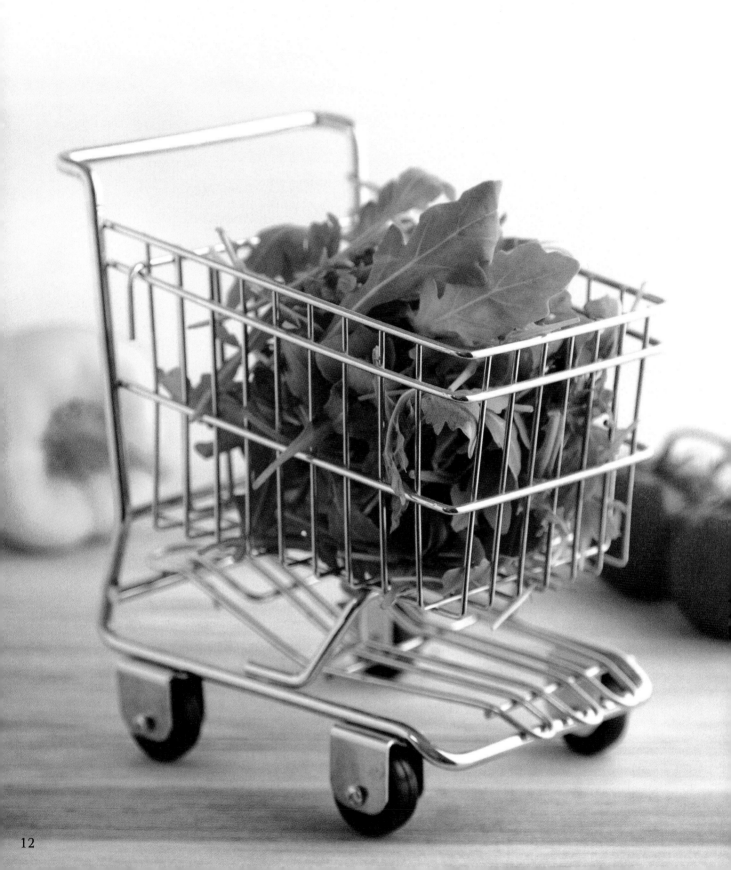

as they measure the ketones in your body. Some blood sugar meters can also measure ketones. Testing is really unnecessary unless you have stalled on losing weight. In that instance, you can use these test strips alongside eliminating specific foods to determine whether a food you are eating is knocking you out of ketosis.

THE LOW-CARB LIFESTYLE

I refer to low-carb as a "lifestyle," as it works best when you eliminate processed carbohydrates completely, without cheating. This is how you achieve ketosis full-time for the maximum benefit.

If you have a lot of weight to lose, I'd highly suggest you go all-in on low-carb. Embrace the lifestyle and eat great tasting, fresh foods every day. It absolutely changed my life and the lives of my family.

FOODS TO AVOID

You can't succeed on low-carb if you don't know which high-carb foods to avoid. Refined grains, sugars, and starches— otherwise known as "the white stuff"— are not a part of a low-carb lifestyle. This includes:

- Flour and all wheat products (bread, pasta, cereal, crackers)
- Sugar (all types, including honey and maple syrup)
- White potatoes and potato products
- Corn products (including cornstarch)
- High-sugar fruits (bananas, mangos, grapes, watermelon, etc.)
- Fruit juice
- Beans
- Milk (cream is fine, but milk has more lactose, which is a form of sugar)

SHOPPING SMART

When grocery shopping, the best rule of thumb is to shop the outer aisles of the store. This is where all of the fresh, naturally low-carb foods are located. The meat, dairy, and produce sections should be your main focus when shopping, as you avoid the inner aisles where the processed junk foods are stacked a mile high.

A key to long-term success is to never let temptations into your cart in the first place. If they don't end up being purchased, they don't end up in your pantry, and don't get snacked on! Instead, stock up on low-carb snacks like fresh vegetables, cheese, nuts, and seeds.

READ THE LABELS

No matter how hard I've tried, I can't completely avoid some packaged food items (such as tomato sauce or paste). When buying anything with a nutritional label, always read the ingredients! Food manufacturers hide sugar and starches in just about anything they can. If you can't make something yourself, you should at least be aware of what is in it.

Simply checking the carb counts on the label is usually not enough, as some products can fall below certain levels (especially products with very small serving sizes), and claim they have zero carbohydrates, even if they contain sugar. A good example of this is non-dairy coffee creamers. They are usually pretty low in carbs, yet they usually contain mostly high-fructose corn syrup and partially-hydrogenated vegetable oil— also known as trans-fat.

THE DIFFERENT PLANS

You've probably heard of several low-carb plans over the years, such as Atkins or Paleo. The options can be a bit overwhelming at first; however, most of these plans share at least one basic principle: eating natural foods that are not processed. Because of this, my fresh recipes are a good choice for nearly any low-carb way of life.

It should be noted though that I don't particularly endorse any specific plan. My family started out on Atkins and found out what worked for us as we went along. We never followed any strict set of rules, and likely broke many rules of The Atkins Diet along the way. You can't always reference a 500-page book before you make dinner, nor can you be expected to retain every nuance written out.

The fundamentals of low-carb have been proven to work and they'll always work, whether you are following a popular plan or not. As long as you are eating low-carbohydrate foods that are not processed, you should be on the right track. To go one step further, you'll have even more success if you make sure that you are eating a good amount of protein and fiber with every meal, as these things slow digestion and keep you feeling full and satisfied. The good news is that most naturally low-carb foods just so happen to contain a good amount of protein and fiber.

In this section, I'll give a brief overview of the biggest differences (and similarities) between the most popular low-carb plans. Whether you want to delve deeper into a specific plan—or simply carve your own path as my family did—is up to you.

THE ATKINS DIET

Atkins is a name that has become synonymous with low-carb (in the way that I hope Stella has become synonymous with low-carb recipes). People like to look for the big NEW thing, but The Atkins Diet has worked for countless people and continues to work decades later.

Atkins is all about phases. Phase 1 is known as "Induction" where you are supposed to eat under 20 grams of carbs a day for 2 weeks, focusing on high-fat and high-protein foods. This kickstarts weight loss.

Phase 2 is the "Balancing" phase where you add more types of foods to your diet that are slightly higher in carbs but still natural, and pretty low in the scheme of things. These are foods like fresh berries, carrots, or sweet potatoes (in moderation). This phase is for continued weight loss.

Phases 3 and 4 are about moving your body into maintenance once you've lost the weight.

All of the recipes in this book are suitable for the weight loss phases of The Atkins Diet.

STELLA STYLE

Stella Style is the name that we gave to our way of eating. I don't like to call it a plan, and don't use the term as much anymore to lessen any confusion as to whether it is a plan. It was always my goal that my readers would find what works for them and develop their own "Style," naming it for themselves, to take ownership over their own accomplishments.

If I ever had any rule, it was (and still is), to shop the outer aisles of your grocery store to focus on buying fresh foods.

As my family started on Atkins, Stella Style is closest to Atkins, though we don't like to put an emphasis on counting carbs. As most of my recipes fall somewhere between the "Induction" and "Balancing" (both weight loss) phases of Atkins, we've never seen a reason to count carbs. We are eating the right foods at all times, and that is all that matters.

All you have to do is flip through this book to see which foods you can eat to replicate our way of eating. Everything we eat is in these recipes at least once.

KETOGENIC

Ketogenic is a newly popular term in the low-carb world. Also known as The Keto Diet, these terms are quickly becoming just a new, fancier way, to say "low-carb."

Ketogenic is simply about eating to keep your body in ketosis, burning fat instead of carbohydrates for energy. It's important to keep in mind that that is the goal of all low-carb diets.

As Ketogenic is not as defined as many other plans, you'll find differences in the "plan" from source to source. Many people (not all) who use the term believe in a very high ratio of fat in foods—literally 70% healthy fats for all foods that you consume.

Low-carb diets tend to be high in fat (which is not a bad thing, as it is then burned for energy), but I've never needed to add fat to my diet to keep my body in ketosis.

Typically, Ketogenic plans suggest 20 net carbs a day, much like the Induction phase of Atkins.

All of the recipes in this book are suitable for most forms of a Ketogenic Diet, however, many may be somewhat lower in fat than other Keto cookbooks.

PALEO

Paleo is the least like the other options listed in this section, as it has several more rules. To be honest, it has a lot of rules.

As you may have heard, Paleo is about eating as the cavemen ate, back before we had refined and processed foods. This is why it is a naturally low-carb diet. However, there are further restrictions on foods than most other low-carb diets. On Paleo, you are supposed to also avoid: salt, refined vegetable oil, butter, cream, cheese, and peanuts.

Many of these things are used throughout this book, however, substitutions can be made to make most of my recipes Paleo-friendly. Olive oil can be used in place of butter or vegetable oil. Coconut milk or unsweetened almond milk can be substituted for cream. Other nut butters can be substituted for peanut butter. Finally, salt and cheese can often be omitted entirely.

That said, these are all foods my family ate while losing weight on low-carb and I don't personally see a reason to restrict anything that doesn't affect your health or results.

SWEETEN THINGS UP

As sugar is a carbohydrate, you can't eat low-carb without cutting out all types of real sugar, including sucrose, glucose, corn syrup, high-fructose corn syrup, added fructose, cane juice, cane syrup, and honey. But once you've cut these things out of your diet, you're inevitably still going to want to indulge in something sweet. You're going to have to find a substitution.

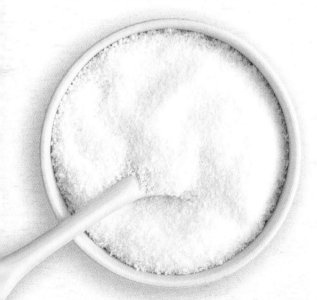

Sugar substitutes are a polarizing topic that has been, and continues to be debated in the news, on the web, and elsewhere. Opinions vary about the different varieties of sugar substitutes, and seem to change too often to keep up with. It is only natural for us to question and, yes, even demand more information on what we put into our bodies. Sugar substitutes often cause people to wonder what is or isn't naturally derived, and for those conscious of eating only natural foods (as we try to do on low-carb), this is wholly understandable.

As a chef, I tend to vote with my palate. It was over a decade ago that I chose to use Splenda as my personal sugar substitute of choice, and have stuck with it ever since. This is simply my own preference due to taste and the fact that it didn't interfere with my weight loss. However, your choice of sugar substitute or "sugar alternative" is left entirely up to you.

THE NEW SUBSTITUTES

There is a remarkable amount of sugar substitutes available in stores today, many of them entirely natural. This luxury simply did not exist back when my family lost the majority of our weight. Back then, Splenda had just hit the shelves and any other alternatives came in either blue or pink packets. These days, you have a plethora of new substitutes to choose from, including erythritol, stevia, monk fruit, and agave nectar, just to name a few. Others are marketed under many different brand names, such as Nevella, Truvia, Stevia Blend, Swerve, Organic Zero, EZ-Sweetz, and Just Like Sugar. The one type of sugar substitute I recommend against is xylitol, as, from what I understand, it can cause digestive discomfort (and is also poisonous to dogs).

DO THEY CAUSE WEIGHT GAIN?

Lately, you may have read that sugar substitutes can actually lead to weight gain. This seems to be the sensational story that is spread around the most right now. My only response to that is that my family consumed

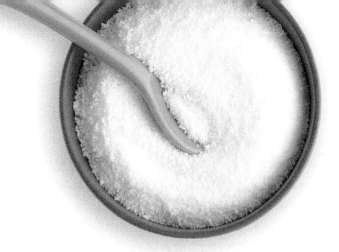

Splenda throughout our weight loss (and we still do), and it never slowed us down! We ate desserts just like those in this book, made of the same ingredients (these exact recipes had not been developed yet) every day of our weight loss, and we had amazing results. Today, we eat the exact desserts in this book to maintain our weight.

It's important to remember that sugar substitutes are among some of the most scrutinized and studied foods on the planet. When in doubt, read these studies and the conclusions of those who publish them, then draw your own conclusion. I made mine long ago and feel comfortable knowing that I've eliminated both sugar and corn syrup from my life.

It is generally well accepted that eating excess sugar can raise your risk for diabetes and other diseases, especially for those who are overweight. The media likes to sensationalize sweeteners, but real sugar (and especially high-fructose corn syrup) is not good for those who are overweight.

MAKE SURE IT'S HEAT STABLE

Regardless of your preference in sweeteners, please check to make sure it is "heat stable" before attempting to bake with it. Aspartame, for instance, (which I do NOT recommend) is not heat stable and will lose its sweetness at a high enough temperature.

The recipes in this book which call for sugar substitute are all measured equal to sugar in order to make them easy to follow, no matter which substitute you prefer. If you are using a brand of sugar substitute that does not measure the same as sugar, simply follow the directions on the package to measure out the correct amount for that particular brand.

Liquid versions of sweeteners listed tend to contain the least amount of carbohydrates, as they require no fillers to add bulk. These also usually measure the least like sugar, so be sure to follow their directions for measuring!

REAL SUGAR...REALLY

Finally, I would like to make one last recommendation. If you have purchased this book with the goal to eat less or no gluten, and not to watch your weight, you can make the choice to use real sugar in my recipes. In the past, I have noticed that many people buy my books purely because of gluten allergies or sensitivities. In this case—if you happen to have no issue with weight, are not at risk for diabetes, and feel comfortable with eating sugar—by all means do so.

Your choice of sweetener is truly your choice to make.

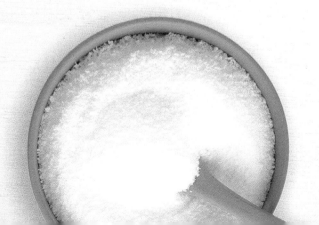

ABOUT THE RECIPES

When I cook, I try to keep things as simple as possible. A recipe can't be "Quick & Easy" if the ingredients are too hard to find, or the directions are impossible to follow. I include subtitles, descriptions, and helpful tips for all of my recipes to help you paint a picture of what you're preparing, and help you prepare it easier. I also include nutritional information to help you make the right choices for your particular diet.

That said, there are some questions you may still have about my recipes, so I've included this section to explain a few unique ingredients, and break down how we've calculated our nutritional information.

UNSALTED BUTTER

The recipes in this book were tested with unsalted butter, however, you can feel free to use salted butter in any savory dish. The impact on flavor will be too minimal to make a difference. That said, we don't recommend using salted butter in our baked goods, as they are truly better without the added salt.

This is a good rule of thumb for most recipes that you'd find anywhere. If it is a savory dish, use the butter you have on hand. If it is a sweet dish or baked good, unsalted butter is usually best.

ALMOND FLOUR

This is the only kind of "flour" we used in the making of this book. It can now be purchased in most grocery stores and is usually found in the baking, organic, or gluten-free sections. Since store-bought almond flour or "almond meal" can be more expensive than preparing it at home, and tends to dry out once baked, we prefer to make our own.

It is incredibly easy to prepare your own almond flour: Simply grind sliced, slivered, or whole raw almonds in a food processor on high for about 3 minutes. Once they've attained a grainy, flour-like consistency, keep stored in an airtight container for up to 1 week on the counter, or for several months in the freezer. Blanched almonds can also be used; these are white and have no hull, making for cleaner "white" flour-like looks, but no difference in flavor. For even smoother consistency, grind small batches of pre-ground almonds through a coffee grinder. You can see an example of both traditional almond flour and blanched almond flour in the pictures on these pages.

While almonds do contain fat (something that white flour does not), this fat happens to be the good (monounsaturated) kind and doesn't deserve to be sneered at. Our baked goods, at first glance, might seem high in fat due to our use of almond flour, though these numbers hold little importance when you take into consideration where the fat comes from. Some studies have even shown that a serving of almonds a day can help boost weight loss.

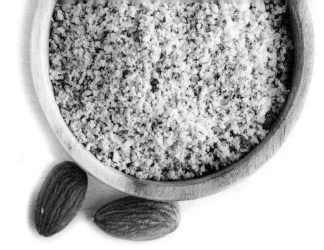

NUTRITIONAL INFORMATION

The nutritional analysis provided in these recipes is meant only as a reference. It was compiled to the best of our ability using nutritional analysis software with an extremely large database of ingredients. Due to variance in the sizes of vegetables, brands of certain foods, or fat content of meat, your calculations may vary.

Calculations are for each serving of the finished dish. Calories in this book were rounded to the nearest 5, and all other amounts were rounded to the nearest .5 of a gram. Optional garnishes or variations were not included in the calculations. Recipes that include the use of another recipe (such as frosting for a cake) already include the nutritional information for the additional recipe as part of the overall dish.

Though we have provided this nutritional information, our family has always made it a point to not count each and every gram of carbohydrates or calories. It is our belief that if you stock your home full of great natural foods and do your best to not "cheat," you'll be eating well enough to see results. I've found that, for many people, counting carbs can lead you to eat worse when trying to save up or "bank" those extra carbs in order

to eat something you probably shouldn't be eating at all. Starving yourself all day to eat an entire pie before bedtime has and never will be a good choice.

We suggest you set yourself free from those numbers altogether, and eat only what is essential for success. Yeah, we know, we know, it is a tough urge to let go of, but trust us—it'll do wonders for your sanity! Get too caught up with counting, and eventually you'll find yourself doing long division on the walls.

NET CARBS

You will notice a number labeled "Net Carbs" in our nutritional information. Net carbs are the carbohydrates that are actually absorbed by your body—the ones that actually affect your blood sugar levels. If you are counting carbs, net carbs are the ones to count.

Our net carbs are determined only by subtracting fiber from the total carbohydrates in the recipe, as fiber does not get absorbed. Food products and other books subtract other things, such as "sugar alcohols," but we ONLY subtract fiber to come up with our net carbs.

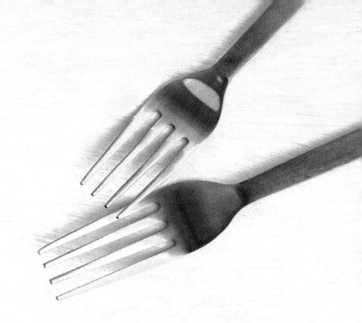

MY TWO-DAY CHALLENGE

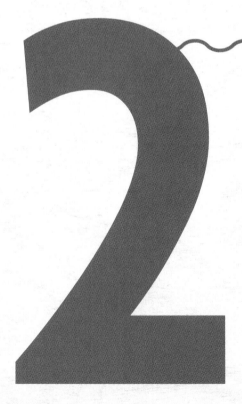

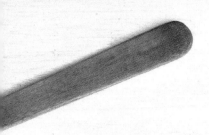

MY TWO-DAY CHALLENGE

While I've already established that low-carb works best when it simply becomes your everyday way of eating—your lifestyle—with your body in a state of ketosis and burning fat, I'd now like to issue a challenge, something completely different for those people who can't quite break their reliance on carbohydrates. My Two-Day Challenge has been issued for those who have tried, but failed, or those who have never had the determination to try in the first place.

A TRIAL RUN

Consider this a trial run, a "try it before you buy it" plan towards success. It's walking before you run…baby steps into the world of eating fresh, naturally low-carb foods. Processed foods are addicting, with a cocktail of carbs, sugar, and salt that hit the pleasure centers of the brain. Sugar (and carbs that convert into sugar in your body) give you a "sugar high" that is hard to resist, even when it can lead to a crash.

BREAKING FREE

My Two-Day Challenge is about breaking that addiction to carbs as you cook and enjoy real food. It's to show how easy and delicious eating low-carb can be; to show you that eating fresh foods can work within your life, and that it can possibly give you more energy, without the crash of those sugar highs.

TRY IT YOURSELF

If you can't go all-in with low-carb, take My Two-Day Challenge by pledging to stop eating processed and refined foods only two days a week. Any two days a week. It could be Saturday and Sunday, when you have less temptations in the work place and more free time to cook; or it could be Monday and Tuesday, to cleanse your body after indulgences of the weekend.

Pick any two days, whether they're subsequent or not, and make the resolution that you'll eat only fresh, naturally low-carb foods on those days. While it won't put your body into a consistent state of ketosis for sustained weight loss, many people eat so many refined carbohydrates that even cutting them out some of the time can make a real difference.

We all have to start somewhere! Start your journey by enjoying recipes from this book just two days a week. Hopefully you'll then find that this is a journey that you can fully commit to. When and if you're ready, you can jump on the low-carb lifestyle full-time, get into that state of ketosis, and feel even better. It's as easy as one, two, days a week!

George Stella

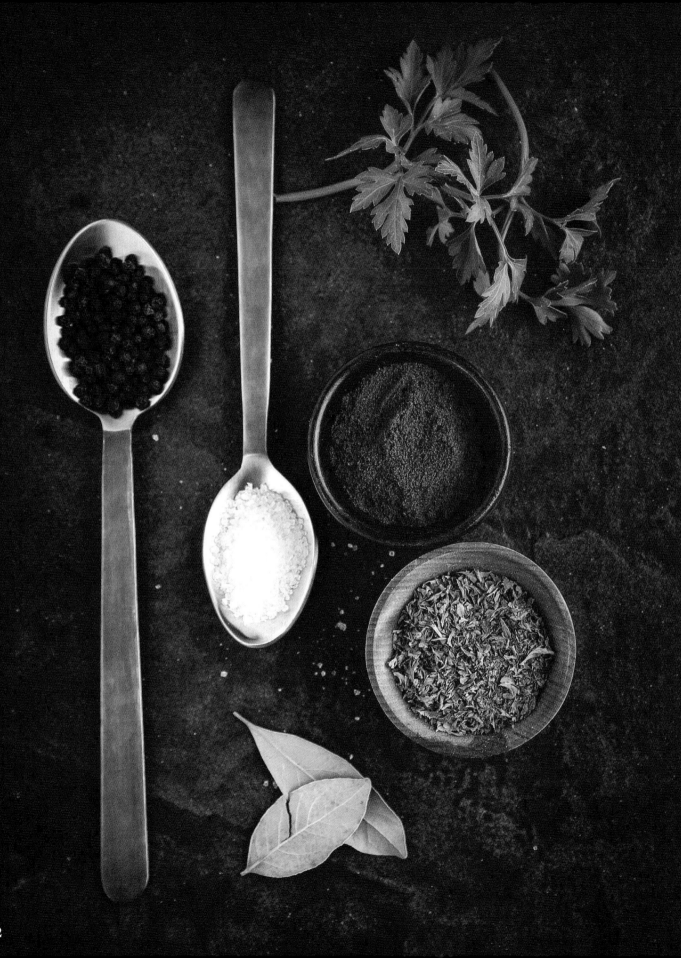

PANTRY LIST

The following is a list of the most commonly used ingredients in this book and in our household. We try to keep most of these ingredients on hand at all times.

SPICE CABINET

- Baking powder
- Bay leaves
- Black pepper
- Cayenne pepper
- Chili powder
- Cider Vinegar
- Cinnamon
- Coconut extract
- Cumin
- Garlic powder
- Italian seasoning

- Nonstick cooking spray
- Olive oil
- Onion powder
- Oregano
- Paprika
- Red wine vinegar
- Smoked paprika
- Thyme
- Vanilla extract
- Vegetable oil

PANTRY

- Almond flour
- Dijon mustard
- Garlic bulbs
- Milled flax seed
- Pecans
- Red onions
- Roasted red peppers

- Spaghetti squash
- Sugar substitute
- Unsweetened baking chocolate
- Unsweetened cocoa powder
- Walnuts
- Worcestershire sauce
- Yellow onions

FRIDGE

- Bacon
- Bell peppers
- Butter
- Cauliflower
- Cilantro
- Cream Cheese
- Eggs

- Fresh herbs
- Half-and-half
- Heavy cream
- Lemons
- Limes
- Parmesan cheese
- Parsley

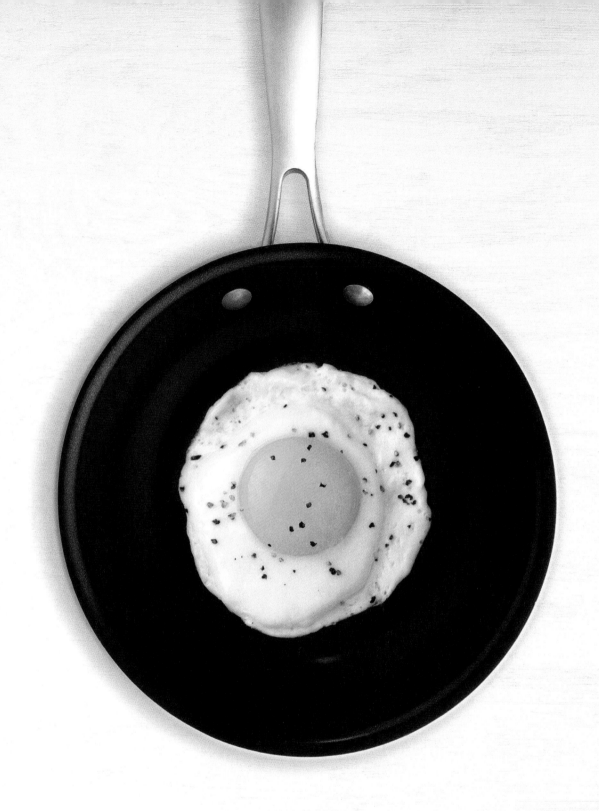

BREAKFAST

~~~~~~~~

QUICK & EASY OMELETS

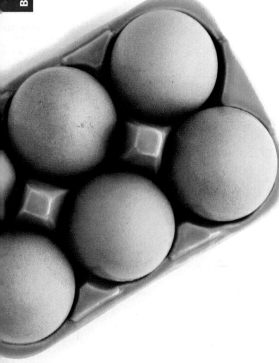

OMELET STARTER RECIPE

EACH RECIPE MAKES 1 OMELET • 1 SERVING

> 2 large eggs
> Pinch salt and black pepper
> 2 teaspoons unsalted butter

1 IN a mixing bowl, whisk eggs with salt and pepper.

2 MELT butter in an 8-inch nonstick pan over medium heat. Add eggs.

3 USE a rubber spatula to move the cooked eggs from the center outward, allowing the uncooked egg to funnel to the center of the pan.

4 ONCE the omelet has mostly set, sprinkle the fillings of your choice over ½ of the surface.

5 USING the rubber spatula, flip the empty half of the omelet over the fillings. Cook for 1 additional minute, just until fillings have warmed through. Top with any toppings or garnishes before serving.

PESTO & FRESH MOZZARELLA OMELET

> 1 tablespoon basil pesto sauce (drop in dollops inside omelet)
> 2 slices fresh mozzarella cheese
> 2 tablespoons fresh diced tomato, to top

Calories: 360 • Fat: 29g • Protein: 22.5g
Total Carbs: 3g – Fiber: 0.5g = **Net Carbs: 2.5g**

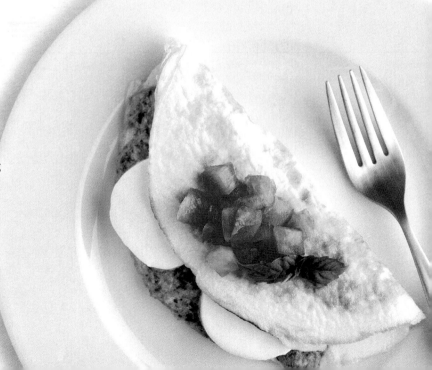

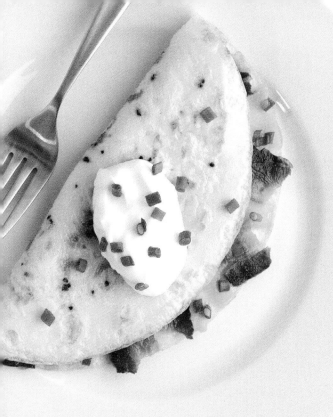

MY FAVORITE OMELET

3 tablespoons shredded Cheddar cheese

2 strips cooked bacon

1 tablespoon chopped chives

1 tablespoon sour cream, to top

Additional chives, to garnish

Calories: 400 • Fat: 34g • Protein: 22.5g
Total Carbs: 1g – Fiber: 0g = **Net Carbs: 1g**

SMOKEHOUSE OMELET

2 slices smoked deli ham, cut into strips

1 ounce smoked Gouda cheese, shredded or thinly sliced

¼ cup arugula, to top

Calories: 355 • Fat: 26g • Protein: 29g
Total Carbs: 1.5g – Fiber: 0g = **Net Carbs: 1.5g**

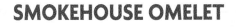

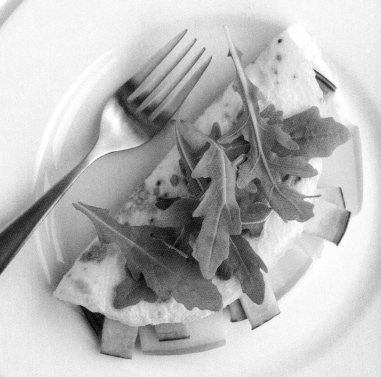

27

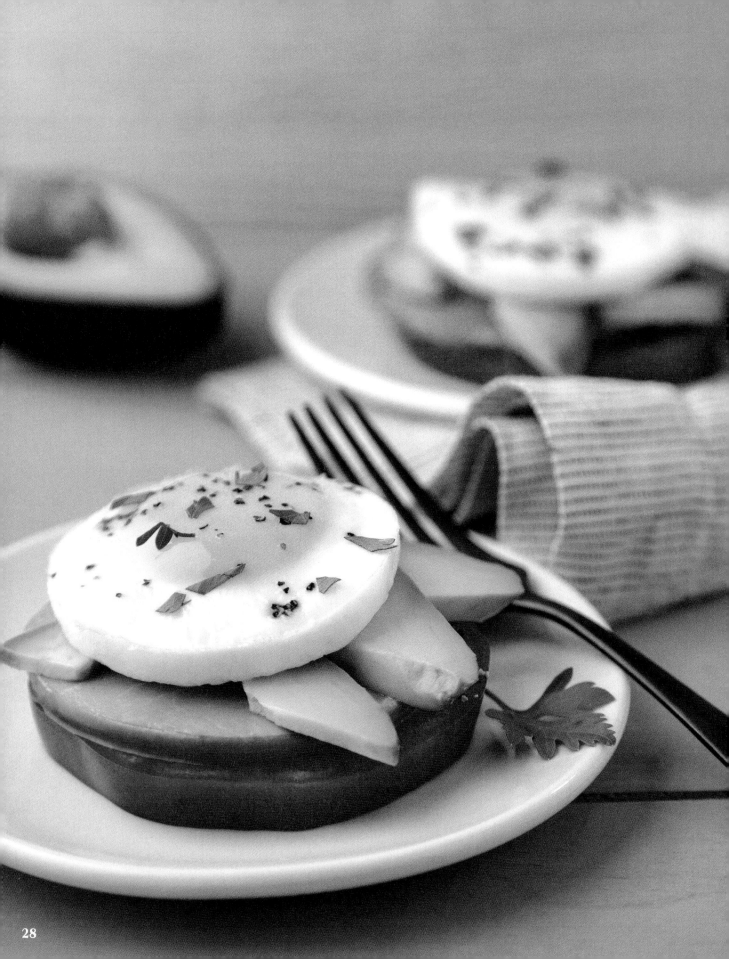

SAN FRAN EGG STACKS

BAKED EGGS OVER TOMATO, CANADIAN BACON, AND AVOCADO

BREAKFAST

These breakfast stacks are piled high with flavor! I like to chill the tomato and avocado before preparing, as it eats like a cold salad topped with a warm egg. Then you break into that yolk and let it become the dressing.

SHOPPING LIST

Nonstick cooking spray

4 large eggs

Salt and black pepper

4 thick slices tomato

4 slices Canadian bacon

1 avocado, thinly sliced

Chopped parsley, for garnish

HELPFUL TIPS

We like to use silicone muffin pans to make these, as you can invert the silicone and pop the cooked eggs right out without any mess.

1 PLACE oven rack in the center position and preheat to 375°F. Spray 4 cups of a 6-cup muffin pan with nonstick cooking spray.

2 CRACK an egg into each prepared muffin cup and lightly season with salt and pepper.

3 BAKE for 10 minutes, or until egg whites are firm but yolks are still soft.

4 As the eggs are baking, prepare 4 serving plates by placing one slice of tomato on each. Season lightly with salt and pepper.

5 TOP the tomato on each plate with a slice of Canadian bacon and an equal amount of the sliced avocado.

6 LET the baked eggs rest in the pan for 1 minute to set before using a rubber spatula or fork to carefully remove. Top each plated stack with a baked egg and garnish with chopped parsley, if desired.

WHAT MAKES IT QUICK & EASY: Baking the eggs gives you the texture and soft yolk of a poached egg, without all of the work…or broken yolks!

Calories: 220 • Fat: 17g • Protein: 13g • Total Carbs: 6g – Fiber: 3.5g = **Net Carbs: 2.5g**

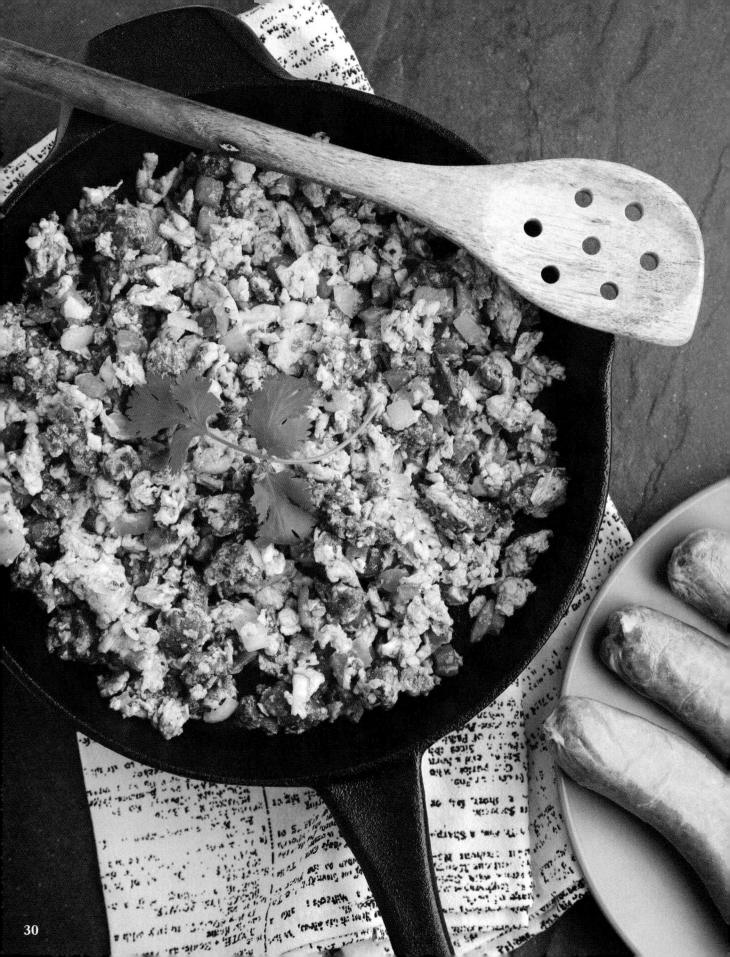

CHORIZO BREAKFAST SKILLET

EGGS SCRAMBLED WITH SPICY SAUSAGE, PEPPERS, AND ONIONS

This simple skillet makes for a full and fulfilling breakfast that packs both flavor and spice. The crumbled chorizo sausage crumbles so finely that it almost mixes right into the scrambled eggs, ensuring that every bite is memorable.

SHOPPING LIST

1 tablespoon olive oil

¼ pound raw chorizo sausage, casings removed (see tip)

¼ cup diced yellow onion

¼ cup diced green bell pepper

6 large eggs, beaten

Salt and black pepper

HELPFUL TIPS

Raw chorizo works best in this recipe as it crumbles and mixes with the egg, however, you can also use smoked (fully cooked) chorizo—Simply slice it thin before adding to the skillet.

1 HEAT oil in a large skillet over medium-high heat.

2 PLACE the sausage in the skillet and crumble it as it browns. Cook until mostly browned, about 5 minutes.

3 ADD the onion and bell pepper to the skillet and sauté 2 minutes, just until onions are translucent. Drain any excess grease.

4 REDUCE heat to medium. Add the eggs to the skillet and scramble together with the chorizo and vegetables. Continue scrambling until eggs are no longer runny, about 5 minutes. Season with salt and pepper to taste before serving.

WHAT MAKES IT QUICK & EASY: This one-skillet breakfast is hearty, yet made with very few ingredients and cooked in only 12 minutes.

Calories: 315 • Fat: 25g • Protein: 20g • Total Carbs: 2g – Fiber: 0g = **Net Carbs: 2g**

BREAKFAST

BUTTER BASTED EGGS

THE MOST FLAVORFUL FRIED EGGS

This simple technique for frying eggs will take you to breakfast nirvana. By basting the top of the eggs with butter and water as the bottoms fry, you get flavor on both sides, without any chance of breaking a yolk or overcooking…I'm looking at you "over-medium."

SHOPPING LIST

1 tablespoon unsalted butter

2 large eggs

Salt and black pepper

2 tablespoons water

HELPFUL TIPS

While this technique works best on gas ranges (as the fire can still make contact with the pan as you tilt it), you can certainly do it on ceramic cooktops, as long as you switch between basting the egg and letting the pan rest on the cooktop to heat up.

1 MELT the butter in a medium nonstick skillet over medium heat.

2 ONCE butter begins to foam, crack two eggs into the pan and lightly season with salt and pepper.

3 ONCE the bottom of the eggs have set, add 2 tablespoons of water to the pan and shake pan from side to side to mix the water with the butter.

4 TILT pan to one side and use a heavy spoon to spoon the water and butter over the uncooked tops of the egg. Continue basting like this until the whites of the egg are firm. Serve immediately.

WHAT MAKES IT QUICK & EASY: It doesn't get much easier than cooking an egg, as long as you know the best way to do it!

Calories: 245 • Fat: 21.5g • Protein: 12.5g • Total Carbs: 0.5g − Fiber: 0g = **Net Carbs: 0.5g**

SNICKERDOODLE MUFFINS

CINNAMON-"SUGAR" MUFFINS

These buttery muffins with cinnamon and sugar substitute taste just like a classic snickerdoodle cookie. It's dessert for breakfast! Or prepare them for actual dessert, and top with my Buttercream Cheese Frosting, recipe page: 194.

SHOPPING LIST

Nonstick cooking spray

½ cup sugar substitute

2 teaspoons ground cinnamon

1¼ cups blanched almond flour

2 teaspoons baking powder

2 large eggs

1 large egg white

2 tablespoons unsalted butter, melted

1 teaspoon vanilla extract

HELPFUL TIPS

You can also use paper liners to line the muffin pan, however you should still spray the insides of the liners with nonstick cooking spray.

1 PLACE oven rack in the center position and preheat to 375°F. Spray a 6-cup muffin pan with nonstick cooking spray.

2 IN a mixing bowl, combine sugar substitute and ground cinnamon. Remove a rounded tablespoon of the mixture and set aside to top the muffins later.

3 STIR the almond flour and baking powder into cinnamon and sugar substitute mixture.

4 IN a separate mixing bowl, beat the eggs, egg white, melted butter, and vanilla extract until frothy.

5 BEAT the dry ingredients into the wet ingredients, until all is combined.

6 FILL the prepared muffin cups with an equal amount of the finished batter, filling each about ⅔ of the way full. Sprinkle the reserved tablespoon of cinnamon and sugar substitute over top of batter in each cup.

7 BAKE for 20–25 minutes, or until centers are firm and springy, and a toothpick inserted into a muffin comes out mostly clean.

8 LET cool for at least 5 minutes before serving.

WHAT MAKES IT QUICK & EASY: Making a muffin batter is even easier than making a cookie batter…plus you get to eat sweets for breakfast!

Calories: 205 • Fat: 17g • Protein: 8g • Total Carbs: 7g – Fiber: 2.5g = **Net Carbs: 4.5g**

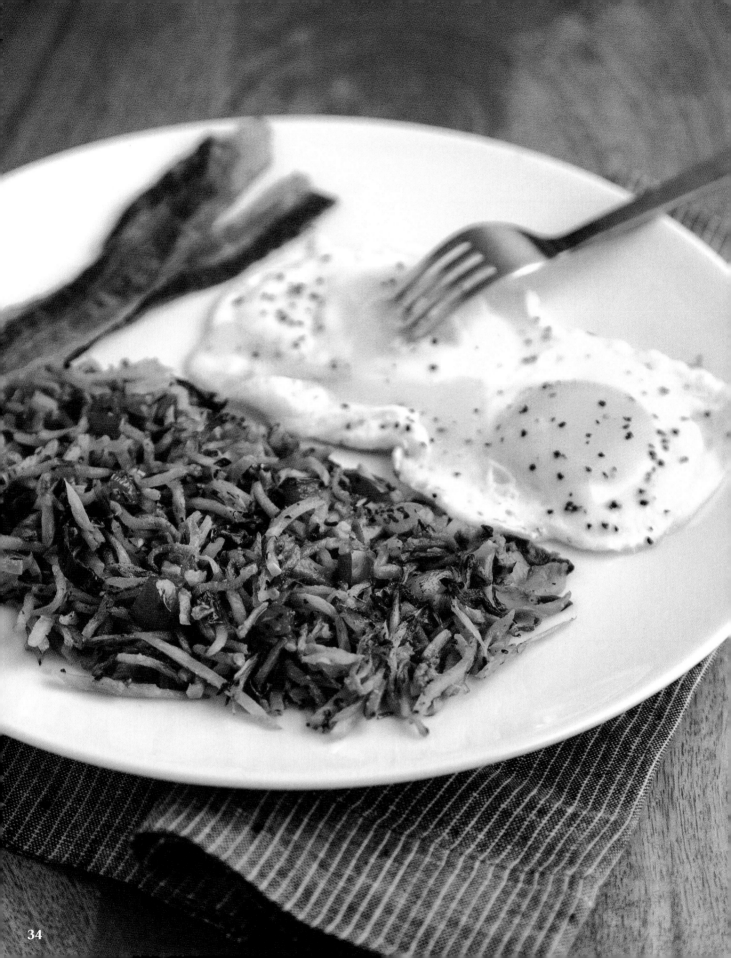

BROCCOLI HASHBROWNS

TOO EASY TO BE TRUE

BREAKFAST

This is one of those recipes you just have to try to understand! It's one thing for me to say that shredded broccoli slaw can taste just like potato hashbrowns, but it's another thing to actually taste it. This is so simple and so good that you won't believe your eyes (when they're seeing broccoli instead of potatoes).

SHOPPING LIST

2 tablespoons unsalted butter

1 (12-ounce) bag shredded broccoli slaw

⅓ cup diced yellow onion

⅓ cup diced red bell pepper

1¼ teaspoons onion powder

½ teaspoon salt

½ teaspoon black pepper

1 HEAT butter in a large skillet over high heat.

2 ONCE butter is melted, add all remaining ingredients to the skillet and stir to combine.

3 COOK, stirring infrequently, about 8 minutes, or until vegetables are well browned.

HELPFUL TIPS

While cooking this over high heat may seem too hot, you really want the broccoli slaw to caramelize, and that needs a very hot pan.

WHAT MAKES IT QUICK & EASY: Using a bag of pre-shredded broccoli slaw mix makes this far easier than shredded traditional potatoes.

Calories: 85 • Fat: 6g • Protein: 2.5g • Total Carbs: 7g − Fiber: 2.5g = **Net Carbs: 4.5g**

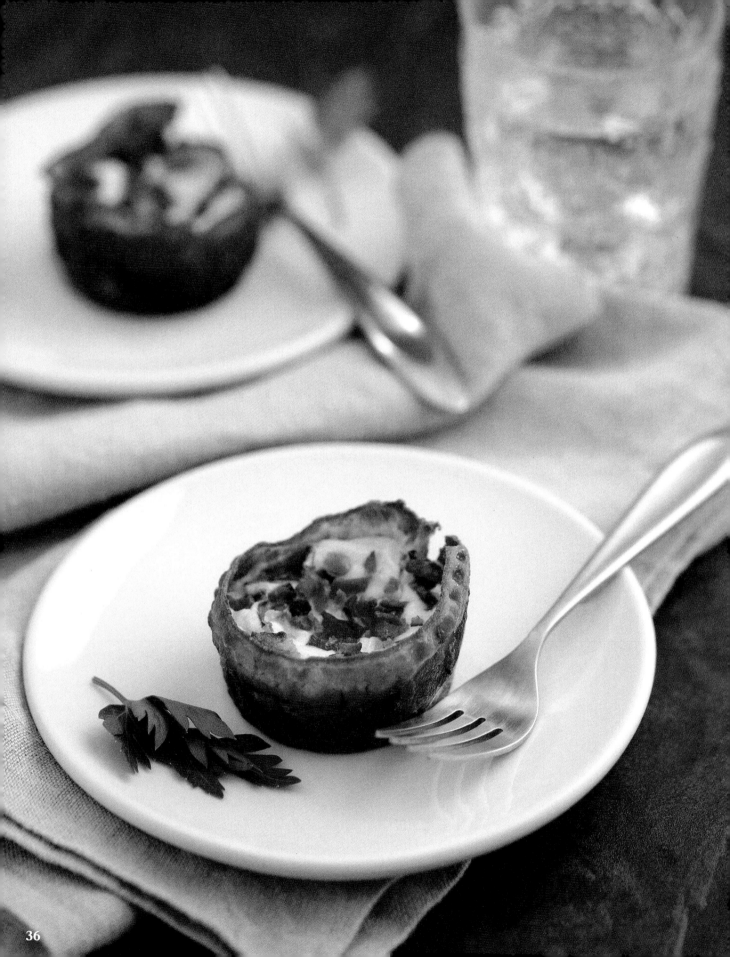

SAVORY BACON CHEESECAKE MINIS
A SAVORY AND UNIQUE BREAKFAST ALTERNATIVE

While these may sound odd at first, you simply need to remove any preconceptions that a cheesecake must be sweet. Think of these bacon-wrapped beauties more like the creamiest quiche you've ever had and you won't be disappointed. They make the absolutely perfect breakfast alternative to a high-carb bagel with cream cheese.

SHOPPING LIST

Nonstick cooking spray

8 strips cooked bacon (see bottom of page)

8 ounces cream cheese, softened

1 large egg

1 tablespoon sugar substitute, optional

⅛ teaspoon onion powder

1 tablespoon finely minced bell pepper

HELPFUL TIPS

I like a small touch of sweetness in these (kind of like using maple flavored bacon), but you can omit the sugar substitute entirely for something that is fully savory.

1 PLACE oven rack in the center position and preheat to 350°F. Spray a 6-cup muffin pan with nonstick cooking spray.

2 CIRCLE the inside of each muffin cup with a strip of cooked bacon. Crumble the remaining two strips of bacon and set aside.

3 ADD the cream cheese, egg, sugar substitute, and onion powder to an electric mixer, and beat on medium speed for 1 minute, just until smooth.

4 SPOON an equal amount of the cream cheese filling into each of the prepared muffin cups, and shake the pan to smooth out.

5 TOP the batter in each cup with an equal amount of the crumbled bacon and minced bell peppers, pressing down lightly to ensure they stick into the batter.

6 BAKE for 30 minutes, or until a toothpick inserted into the center of a cheesecake comes out mostly clean.

7 LET cool for 10 minutes before serving warm, or serve chilled.

WHAT MAKES IT QUICK & EASY: We make these really easy by using the precooked bacon you can buy at the grocery store. It works perfectly!

Calories: 200 • Fat: 18.5g • Protein: 6.5g • Total Carbs: 1.5g − Fiber: 0g = **Net Carbs: 1.5g**

EGG BISCUITS & SAUSAGE GRAVY
A LOW-CARB REINVENTION OF A COUNTRY CLASSIC

Move over biscuits! In this recipe, I top fluffy baked eggs with a classic (and low-carb) sausage gravy. Coarse ground or freshly cracked black pepper is highly recommended, as that is the real secret to a really great white gravy.

SHOPPING LIST

Nonstick cooking spray
4 large eggs
Salt and black pepper

SAUSAGE GRAVY

¼ pound ground breakfast sausage
½ cup heavy cream
½ teaspoon cracked black pepper
¼ teaspoon salt

HELPFUL TIPS

We like to use silicone muffin pans to make the eggs in this recipe, as you can invert the silicone and pop the cooked eggs right out without any mess.

1 PLACE oven rack in the center position and preheat oven to 375°F. Spray 4 cups of a 6-cup muffin pan with nonstick cooking spray.

2 CRACK an egg into each prepared muffin cup, and lightly season with salt and pepper.

3 BAKE for 10 minutes, or until egg whites are firm, but yolks are still soft.

4 As the eggs are baking, prepare the Sausage Gravy. Place a medium skillet over medium-high heat.

5 ADD the breakfast sausage to the skillet, and crumble as it browns. Cook until fully browned, about 5 minutes. Drain excess grease.

6 STIR the heavy cream, pepper, and salt into the browned sausage, and heat just until cream is warmed, about 1 minute.

7 LET the baked eggs rest in the pan for 1 minute to set before using a rubber spatula or fork to carefully remove. Top each egg with a few tablespoons of the Sauasage Gravy before serving.

WHAT MAKES IT QUICK & EASY: By making the Sausage Gravy as the eggs bake, you can cook this entire recipe in only 10 minutes.

Calories: 225 • Fat: 18.5g • Protein: 12g • Total Carbs: 1g − Fiber: 0g = **Net Carbs: 1g**

BANANA PECAN PANCAKES

FLOUR-FREE FLAPJACKS FLAVORED WITH BANANA

This is my favorite method for making reinvented pancakes, as they come out light, fluffy, and sweet enough to eat without syrup. For even more decadence, I like to top mine with a dollop of sugar-free whipped cream.

SHOPPING LIST

4 ounces cream cheese, softened

4 large eggs

⅓ cup sugar substitute

½ teaspoon banana extract

Nonstick cooking spray

⅓ cup chopped pecans

HELPFUL TIPS

While you can also add the chopped pecans to the pancakes themselves before you flip them to cook on the second side, I find that they hold together better when using the pecans as a topping.

1 IN a food processor or blender, pulse cream cheese, eggs, sugar substitute, and banana extract until a smooth batter is formed.

2 SPRAY an 8-inch nonstick pan with nonstick cooking spray, and place over medium heat.

3 ONCE the pan is hot, add 2 tablespoons of the batter and tilt the pan from side to side until the mix almost coats the entire surface of the pan.

4 COOK for 2 minutes before flipping to cook for 1 additional minute, or until golden brown on both sides.

5 REPEAT using additional nonstick cooking spray until all batter has been used up.

6 TOP each 2-pancake serving with a sprinkling of chopped pecans before serving.

WHAT MAKES IT QUICK & EASY: Mixing the batter in the blender makes incorporating the cream cheese and eggs as simple as flipping a switch.

Calories: 250 • Fat: 22g • Protein: 9.5g • Total Carbs: 4.5g – Fiber: 1g = **Net Carbs: 3.5g**

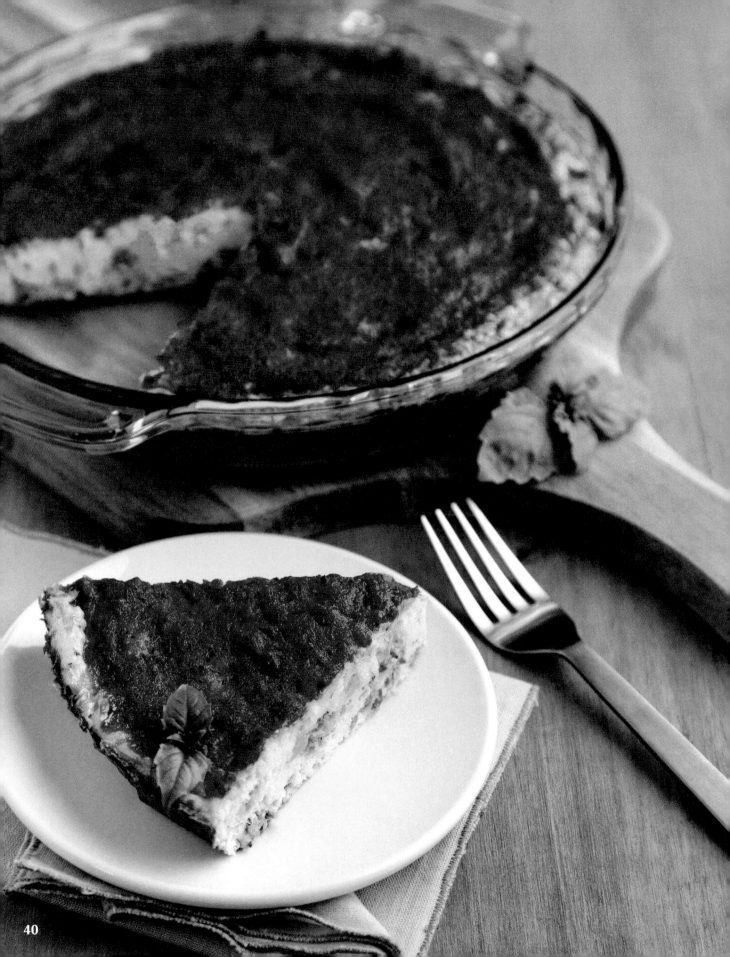

CHICAGO DEEP DISH QUICHE

IT'S PIZZA FOR BREAKFAST!

Grab a slice of this true reinvention of Chicago-style deep dish pizza. You've got all the elements you'd find in The Windy City—sausage, peppers, and loads of cheese—only baked into a quiche rather than a crust. You even have the sauce on the top, just like the real deal.

SHOPPING LIST

Nonstick cooking spray

8 ounces ground Italian sausage, casings removed

⅔ cup diced yellow onion

⅔ cup diced bell pepper (any color)

2 cups shredded mozzarella cheese

8 large eggs

¼ cup heavy cream

¾ teaspoon salt

½ teaspoon black pepper

¼ teaspoon Italian seasoning

⅔ cup pizza sauce (see tip)

HELPFUL TIPS

I found that my local store-brand of pizza sauce had no added sugars. Any brand of pasta sauce without added sugar can be used.

1 PREHEAT oven to 350°F. Spray a 9-inch deep dish pie plate with nonstick cooking spray.

2 ADD Italian sausage, onion, and bell pepper to a skillet over medium-high heat, and cook until well browned.

3 DRAIN any excess grease from the browned sausage, and then transfer to the prepared pie plate. Top with the mozzarella cheese.

4 IN a mixing bowl, whisk together the eggs, heavy cream, salt, pepper, and Italian seasoning.

5 POUR the egg mixture over the sausage and cheese in the pie plate.

6 BAKE for 40 minutes, just until mostly set.

7 SPREAD the pizza sauce over the top of the quiche, and bake an additional 15 minutes. Let rest 5 minutes before serving warm.

WHAT MAKES IT QUICK & EASY: While this is the longest recipe to make in this chapter, it is still far less complicated than making an actual deep dish pizza!

Calories: 240 · Fat: 16g · Protein: 18.5g · Total Carbs: 4.5g – Fiber: 1g = **Net Carbs: 3.5g**

BREAKFAST

GREEN EGGS & HAM SCRAMBLE

EGGS SCRAMBLED WITH AVOCADO, GREEN ONIONS, AND HAM

There's no more important meal to prepare in one pan than breakfast…I mean, who wants a sink full of dishes that early in the morning? Now I know that many chefs have played off Dr. Seuss for "green" egg recipes over the years, but I couldn't resist joining in. You've got avocado and ham scrambled into the eggs; there was simply no better name!

SHOPPING LIST

2 teaspoons olive oil

⅔ cup diced or cubed ham

5 large eggs, beaten

¼ teaspoon salt

¼ teaspoon black pepper

½ avocado, chopped

2 tablespoons sliced green onions

HELPFUL TIPS

The best way to check an avocado for ripeness is to pull the stem out. If it gives way easily and shows green, you've got a ripe avocado. If it takes a little effort and shows yellow, it is not yet ripe.

1 HEAT oil in a large skillet over medium-high heat.

2 PLACE the ham in the skillet, and cook until lightly browned, about 4 minutes.

3 REDUCE heat to medium. Add the eggs to the skillet, and scramble together with the ham. Continue scrambling until eggs are only slightly runny, about 4 minutes.

4 STIR in avocado and green onions, and cook for 2 additional minutes, or until eggs are mostly firm. Season with any additional salt and pepper to taste before serving.

WHAT MAKES IT QUICK & EASY: If using pre-diced ham, you'll only have to chop avocado and green onion to make this fulfilling breakfast.

Calories: 275 • Fat: 20g • Protein: 20.5g • Total Carbs: 4.5g − Fiber: 2.5g = **Net Carbs: 2g**

SPINACH & ARTICHOKE FRITTATA
TOPPED WITH SHREDDED PARMESAN CHEESE

Frittatas make the perfect breakfast for feeding a few people with very little effort. I make them all the time, and this Spinach & Artichoke Frittata is one of my personal favorites. It's a classic combination of flavors that goes great with the light and fluffy eggs.

SHOPPING LIST

1 tablespoon olive oil

2 cups fresh spinach leaves

½ teaspoon minced garlic

6 large eggs

¼ teaspoon salt

¼ teaspoon black pepper

⅛ teaspoon baking powder

⅔ cup quartered artichoke hearts (canned or jarred), drained

⅔ cup shredded Parmesan cheese

HELPFUL TIPS

⅔ cup of frozen chopped spinach can be used in place of the fresh spinach in this recipe.

1 PREHEAT oven to 325°F.

2 HEAT the olive oil in a large ovenproof skillet over medium heat.

3 ADD the spinach and garlic to the skillet, and sauté just until the spinach has cooked down, about 2 minutes. Drain any excess liquid.

4 IN a mixing bowl, whisk together the eggs, salt, pepper, and baking powder. Pour over the vegetables in the skillet.

5 USING a rubber spatula, gently push the cooked egg from one side of the pan to the other to allow more of the raw egg to reach the bottom of the pan. Continue doing this until the top of the eggs are only slightly runny.

6 ARRANGE the artichoke hearts over the runny eggs, and then top all with Parmesan cheese.

7 BAKE for 10 minutes, or until eggs begin to puff up. Serve immediately.

WHAT MAKES IT QUICK & EASY: This makes for an upscale breakfast using only one skillet.

Calories: 220 · Fat: 16g · Protein: 16.5g · Total Carbs: 5g − Fiber: 2g = **Net Carbs: 3g**

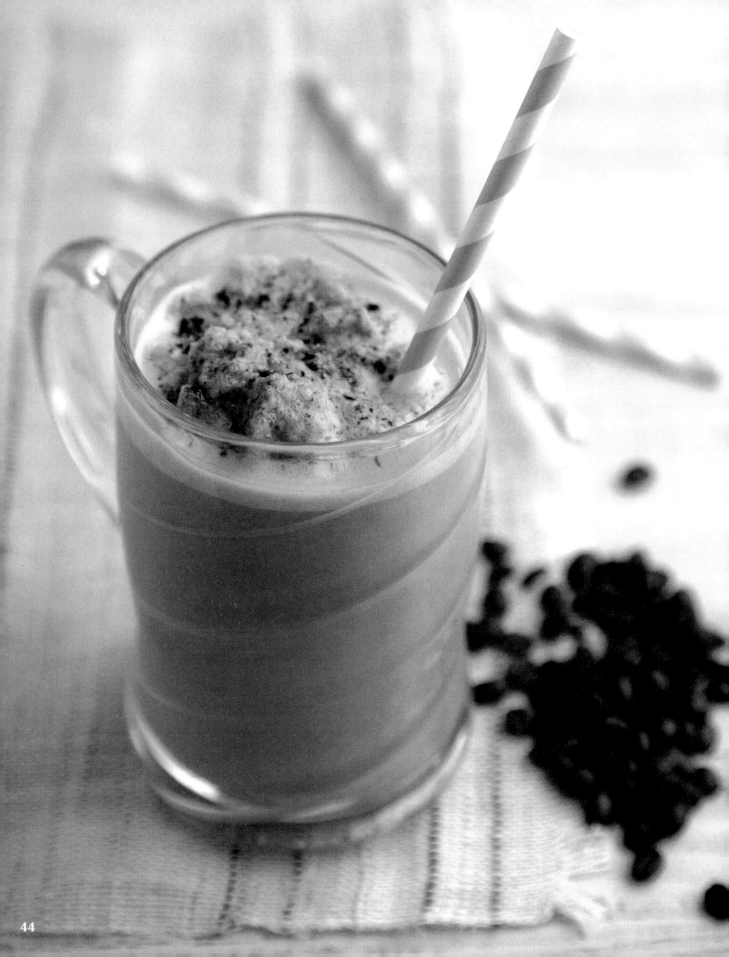

MOCHA BREAKFAST SHAKE
A DAIRY-FREE COFFEE SHOP PICK-ME-UP

Don't be scared off by the tofu in this creamy breakfast shake…I assure you that it adds no flavor whatsoever. What it does add is protein and a silky texture that will have you thinking that there's got to be dairy in this drink.

SHOPPING LIST

1¼ cups unsweetened almond milk

8 ounces silken tofu

3 tablespoons sugar substitute

3 teaspoons instant coffee granules

1 teaspoon cocoa powder

¼ teaspoon vanilla extract

1 cup ice cubes

1   ADD all ingredients, except ice, to a blender and blend until smooth.

2   ADD ice to the blender and blend well. Serve immediately, garnished with a sprinkling of additional instant coffee granules or cocoa powder, if desired.

HELPFUL TIPS

Silken tofu is usually sold in the refrigerated section of the produce department, near the vegetarian meat and cheese substitutes.

WHAT MAKES IT QUICK & EASY: This one-blender breakfast is easily whipped up in less than 5 minutes.

Calories: 90 • Fat: 4.5g • Protein: 7g • Total Carbs: 5g − Fiber: 0.5g = **Net Carbs: 4.5g**

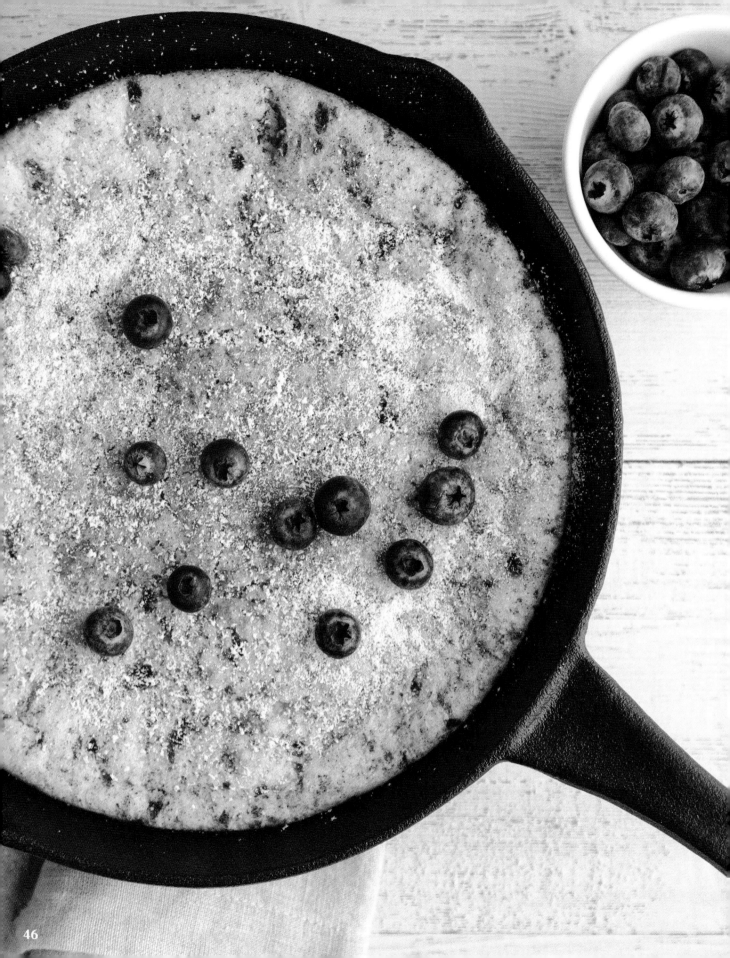

"DUTCH BABY" PANCAKE
A GIANT OVEN-BAKED PANCAKE

While I don't know how this eggy, puffed-up pancake became known as a "Dutch Baby," I do know that my low-carb reinvention makes a great family breakfast. With the flavors of maple and cinnamon baked in, you may find that this tastes more like French Toast than a pancake, but that's not a bad thing. It has so much flavor that you don't even need syrup!

SHOPPING LIST

4 large eggs

⅓ cup half-and-half

⅓ cup blanched almond flour

⅓ cup sugar substitute

2 tablespoons unsalted butter, melted

1 teaspoon baking powder

¾ teaspoon ground cinnamon

½ teaspoon maple extract

Nonstick cooking spray

HELPFUL TIPS

Always be sure to wear oven mitts when handling the baked skillet in this recipe!

1 PLACE a cast-iron skillet on the oven's center rack and preheat oven to 400°F, letting the skillet preheat with it.

2 IN a mixing bowl, whisk together all ingredients, except nonstick cooking spray, to create a batter.

3 ONCE preheated, spray the skillet with nonstick cooking spray. Pour batter into the greased skillet.

4 BAKE for 17–20 minutes, just until the pancake has puffed up and begins to brown on the top.

5 SERVE sprinkled with additional sugar substitute, if desired.

WHAT MAKES IT QUICK & EASY: It's always easier to make one giant pancake to share, rather than several batches of smaller pancakes!

Calories: 210 • Fat: 17.5g • Protein: 9g • Total Carbs: 5.5g − Fiber: 1g = **Net Carbs: 4.5g**

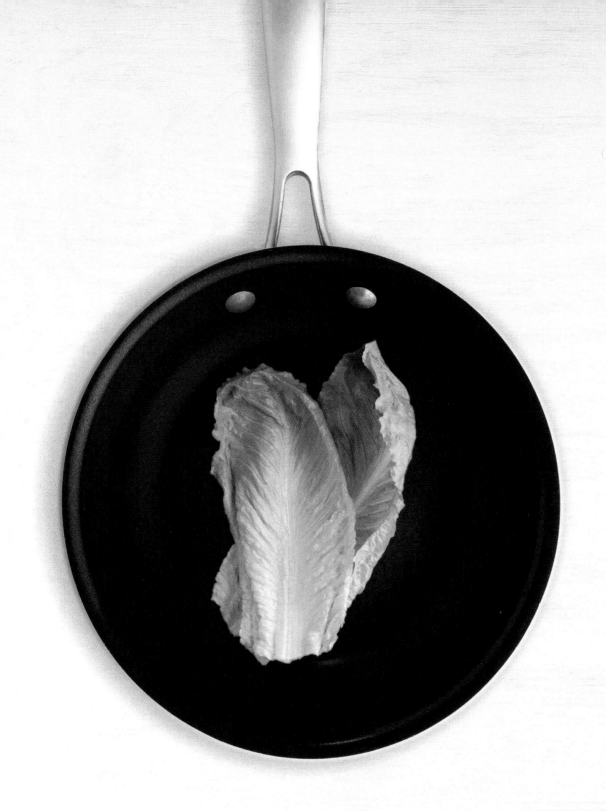

LUNCH

QUICK & EASY SALAD DRESSINGS

HONEY DIJON DRESSING

MAKES ABOUT 7 (2-TABLESPOON) SERVINGS

½ cup heavy cream

¼ cup country-style or stone-ground Dijon mustard

2 tablespoons yellow mustard

2 tablespoons sugar substitute

½ teaspoon dried rosemary

1 In a mixing bowl, whisk together all ingredients.

2 Store covered and refrigerated for up to 7 days.

Calories: 40 • Fat: 4g • Protein: 1g
Total Carbs: 1g – Fiber: 0g = **Net Carbs: 1g**

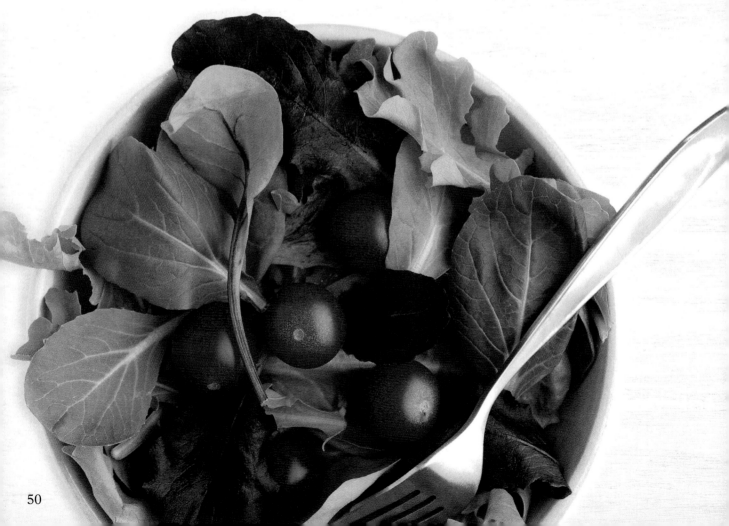

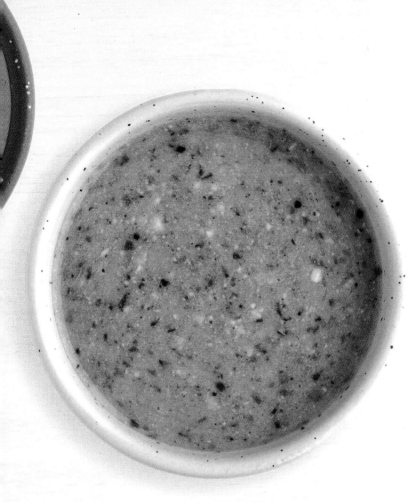

GREEK VINAIGRETTE

MAKES ABOUT 8 (2-TABLESPOON) SERVINGS

⅓ cup red wine vinegar

¼ finely crumbled feta cheese

1 tablespoon minced garlic

1½ teaspoons dried oregano

1 teaspoon Dijon mustard

½ teaspoon sugar substitute

½ teaspoon pepper

¼ teaspoon salt

½ cup extra-virgin olive oil

1 IN a mixing bowl, whisk together all ingredients, except olive oil.

2 WHILE constantly whisking, slowly add the olive oil a little at a time, until all is incorporated.

3 STORE covered and refrigerated for up to 7 days. Stir or shake before serving.

Calories: 130 • Fat: 14g • Protein: 1g
Total Carbs: 1g – Fiber: 0g = **Net Carbs: 1g**

BLUE CHEESE DRESSING

MAKES ABOUT 8 (2-TABLESPOON) SERVINGS

½ cup blue cheese crumbles

⅓ cup heavy cream

⅓ cup sour cream

½ teaspoon Worcestershire sauce

½ teaspoon sugar substitute

½ teaspoon pepper

¼ teaspoon garlic powder

¼ teaspoon salt

1 IN a mixing bowl, whisk together all ingredients.

2 FOR best flavor, use a fork to mash larger chunks of the blue cheese into the dressing.

3 STORE covered and refrigerated for up to 7 days.

Calories: 65 • Fat: 6g • Protein: 1.5g
Total Carbs: 1g – Fiber: 0g = **Net Carbs: 1g**

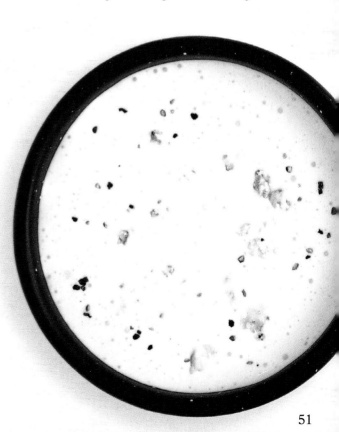

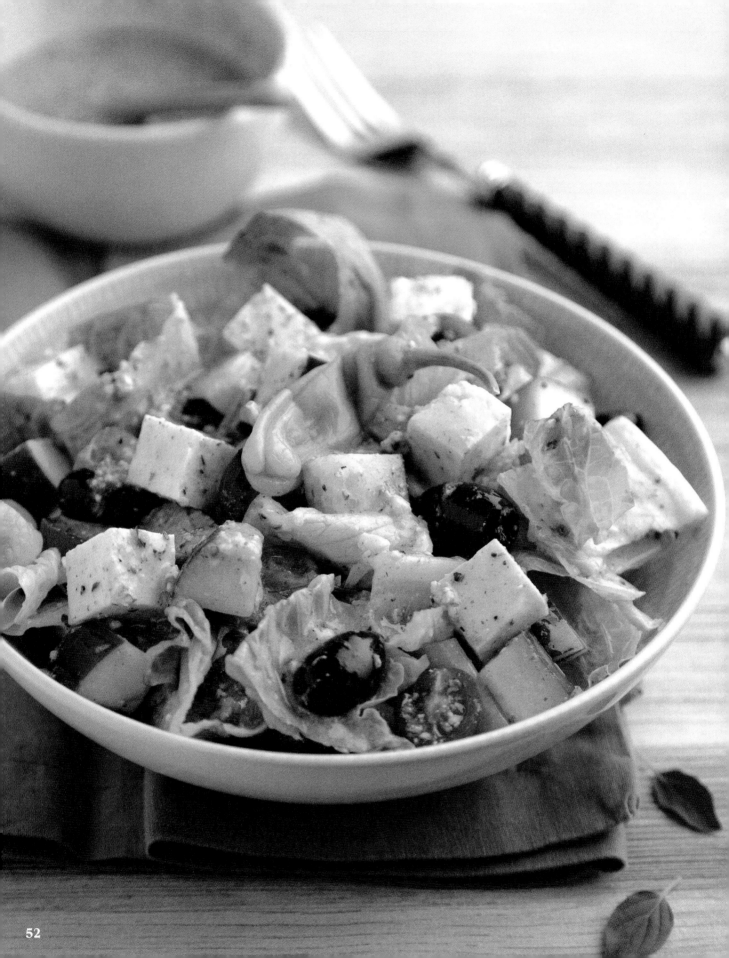

CHOPPED GREEK SALAD

A CLASSIC GREEK SALAD, ALL MIXED UP

Greek salads are loaded with vibrant and flavorful low-carb ingredients! In this recipe, I've chopped and tossed those flavors in my delicious Greek Vinaigrette, recipe page: 51. Nutritional information includes the Greek Vinaigrette dressing.

SHOPPING LIST

1 (10-ounce) bag chopped romaine lettuce

1 small cucumber, chopped

⅔ cup cherry tomatoes, halved

½ cup pitted Kalamata olives, drained

4 ounces feta cheese, diced or crumbled

3 tablespoons diced red onion

¼ cup Greek Vinaigrette, recipe page: 51

Pickled pepperoncini peppers, for garnish

1 PLACE lettuce, cucumber, tomatoes, Kalamata olives, feta, and onion in a large salad bowl.

2 POUR Greek Vinaigrette over top and toss to combine.

3 SERVE immediately, garnished with pepperoncini peppers, if desired.

HELPFUL TIPS

You can chop 2 heads of romaine hearts in place of the bagged lettuce.

WHAT MAKES IT QUICK & EASY: If you purchase small tomatoes that don't need halving, and pre-crumbled feta, you'll only need to chop the cucumber and onion.

Calories: 190 • Fat: 16g • Protein: 5.5g • Total Carbs: 8g − Fiber: 2g = **Net Carbs: 6g**

HARVEST SALAD

WITH CHICKEN, SPINACH, RASPBERRIES AND PECANS

This vibrant spinach salad is the perfect combination of sweet and savory ingredients to serve alongside my Honey Dijon Dressing, recipe page: 50. This makes 2 very large lunch portions, with a full chicken breast on each salad.

SHOPPING LIST

4 cups baby spinach leaves

⅓ cup shelled pecan halves

⅓ cup fresh raspberries

¼ cup thinly sliced red onion

12 ounces sliced or chopped chicken breast (see tip)

Honey Dijon Dressing, recipe page: 50, if desired

1 PLACE spinach in two individual serving bowls.

2 TOP the spinach in each bowl with an equal amount of the pecans, raspberries, and sliced red onion.

3 TOP each salad with an equal amount of the cooked chicken.

4 SERVE immediately, alongside my Honey Dijon Dressing, if desired.

HELPFUL TIPS

For the best presentation you can top each salad with a full (6-ounce) chicken breast that has been cooked and sliced (but arranged in the original shape of the chicken breast before slicing).

WHAT MAKES IT QUICK & EASY: I like to grill extra chicken breasts when I'm grilling for dinner—that way I can easily prepare salads like this the next day.

Calories: 335 • Fat: 16.5g • Protein: 43g • Total Carbs: 8.5g − Fiber: 5g = **Net Carbs: 3.5g**

CREAM OF MUSHROOM SOUP
MADE WITH AN ENTIRE POUND OF FRESH MUSHROOMS

For most people, their only experience with Cream of Mushroom Soup is with the condensed, canned version—but I promise you that it can be far, far better than that! Possibly more than any other ingredient, the difference between canned and fresh mushrooms is night and day. While it could never be as easy as opening a can, the robust flavor of this soup is well worth the extra 10 minutes of prep time.

SHOPPING LIST

2 tablespoons unsalted butter

1 pound baby bella mushrooms, chopped

3 tablespoons minced yellow onion

1 tablespoon minced garlic

3 cups beef stock

½ cup heavy cream

2 sprigs fresh thyme

2 bay leaves

½ teaspoon black pepper

6 ounces cream cheese

Salt

1 HEAT butter in a large pot over medium-high heat, until sizzling.

2 PLACE mushrooms in the hot pot and let cook, without moving, until browned, about 4 minutes.

3 STIR in onion and garlic and sauté for 3 minutes.

4 STIR in beef stock, heavy cream, thyme, bay leaves, and pepper. Bring up to a simmer.

5 REDUCE heat to medium-low, and let simmer 10 minutes.

6 REMOVE from heat and stir in cream cheese. Remove thyme and bay leaves, and season with salt to taste before serving.

HELPFUL TIPS

For an even more concentrated mushroom flavor, and a slightly thicker soup, you can transfer half of the mushrooms and 1 cup of the soup to a blender after cooking, and purée until smooth. Then stir this purée back into the full pot of soup.

WHAT MAKES IT QUICK & EASY: Soups like this one usually start by cooking a roux with butter and flour; however, I use cream cheese to thicken the soup the low-carb way!

Calories: 290 • Fat: 26.5g • Protein: 6.5g • Total Carbs: 8.5g − Fiber: 2g = **Net Carbs: 6g**

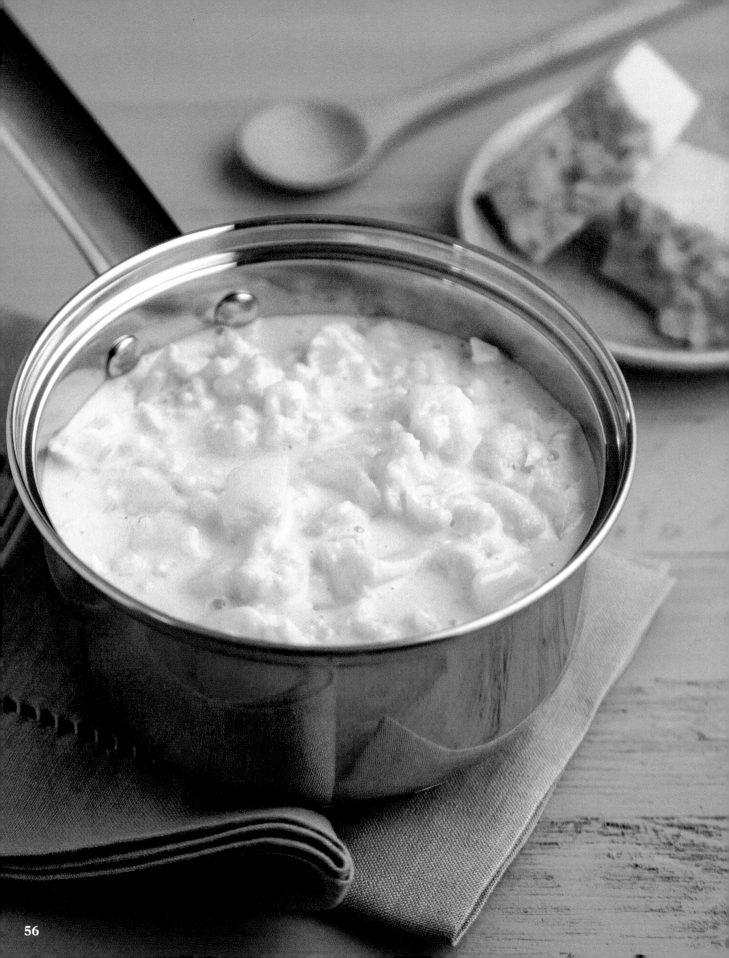

STOVETOP MOCK MAC & CHEESE

A FAN-FAVORITE, MADE EASIER

My original recipe for Mock Mac has been pleasing families for over a decade, but I've now made it even easier. In this all-new version, I skip the oven, and make it entirely on the stove, without sacrificing the flavor or texture that people expect—in fact, I think it is even creamier than the original!

LUNCH

SHOPPING LIST

1 head cauliflower

2/3 cup heavy cream

3/4 teaspoon ground mustard

1/2 teaspoon salt

1/4 teaspoon garlic powder

1 1/4 cups sharp Cheddar cheese

4 slices deluxe American cheese

HELPFUL TIPS

I always buy American cheese labeled "deluxe," as it not only tastes better, but has slightly less carbs from milk sugar.

1   CHOP cauliflower into small pieces, stem and all. Discard leaves.

2   BOIL or steam chopped cauliflower for 10 minutes, until very tender. Drain well.

3   TRANSFER drained cauliflower to a sauce pot over medium heat, and add heavy cream, mustard, salt, and garlic powder.

4   STIRRING frequently, bring the heavy cream in the pot to a simmer. Let simmer for 5 minutes.

5   REMOVE pot from heat and stir in Cheddar and American cheeses, stirring until well combined. Let stand 1 minute to thicken before serving.

WHAT MAKES IT QUICK & EASY: Using the American cheese helps bind the Cheddar cheese with the heavy cream, so that it is easier to mix without the sauce separating.

Calories: 310 · Fat: 25g · Protein: 14.5g · Total Carbs: 7g − Fiber: 3g = **Net Carbs: 4g**

CREAMY PESTO CHICKEN SALAD

A PICNIC SALAD WITH FRESH BASIL AND WHOLE PINE NUTS

This chunky mayonnaise-based chicken salad has all the flavors of pesto, without the blending. Toasted pine nuts are left whole to add a bit of texture to the final picnic salad. For the quickest and easiest starting point, simply purchase a cooked rotisserie chicken from the grocery store, and you'll be on your way to chicken salad that can't be beat.

SHOPPING LIST

DRESSING

⅓ cup mayonnaise

3 tablespoons finely chopped fresh basil

3 tablespoons grated Parmesan cheese

2 tablespoons water

1 tablespoon extra-virgin olive oil

1 teaspoon lemon juice

¼ teaspoon salt

¼ teaspoon black pepper

SALAD

2 cups shredded or diced cooked chicken breast

3 tablespoons toasted pine nuts (see tip)

1 ADD all Dressing ingredients to a large mixing bowl, and whisk to combine.

2 ADD the Salad ingredients into the Dressing, folding until well coated.

3 FOR best flavor, cover and refrigerate for at least 1 hour before serving.

HELPFUL TIPS

To toast pine nuts, simply bake in a 375°F oven for 6–8 minutes, just until golden brown and fragrant.

WHAT MAKES IT QUICK & EASY: This can be made into a quick lunch by serving over a bed of lettuce or spinach with sliced tomatoes.

Calories: 340 • Fat: 25.5g • Protein: 27.5g • Total Carbs: 1g – Fiber: 0g = **Net Carbs: 1g**

BETTER BUTTER BURGERS
BASIC BURGERS PAN-SEARED IN BUTTER

There's nothing better than a burger seared in butter! Not only is it far faster than waiting for the grill to preheat, the butter also creates a beautiful browned crust on the patty that you can't get any other way. Montreal steak seasoning (found in the spice aisle of the grocery store) is my favorite for seasoning burgers, and it couldn't be any easier.

SHOPPING LIST

2 tablespoons unsalted butter

4 (¼-pound) ground beef patties

Montreal steak seasoning

Lettuce, if desired

Burger toppings, if desired

HELPFUL TIPS

You can choose to form your own patties, or buy them pre-formed at the store; however, I don't suggest you buy them frozen. Fresh is best with ground beef.

1 HEAT butter in a large skillet over medium-high heat, until sizzling.

2 GENEROUSLY season both sides of the burger patties.

3 PLACE seasoned burgers in the skillet, and cook for 3 minutes on each side for medium-rare to medium. Cook for 4–5 minutes on each side for medium to medium-well.

4 SERVE on a bed of lettuce, topped with your favorite burger toppings, if desired.

5 FOR Cheeseburgers: Top with cheese 1 minute before burgers have finished cooking, and cover pan to trap the heat in, melting the cheese.

WHAT MAKES IT QUICK & EASY: If you buy pre-formed, but still fresh, ground beef patties, you can be cooking these burgers in seconds!

Calories: 330 • Fat: 24g • Protein: 27.5g • Total Carbs: 0g – Fiber: 0g = **Net Carbs: 0g**

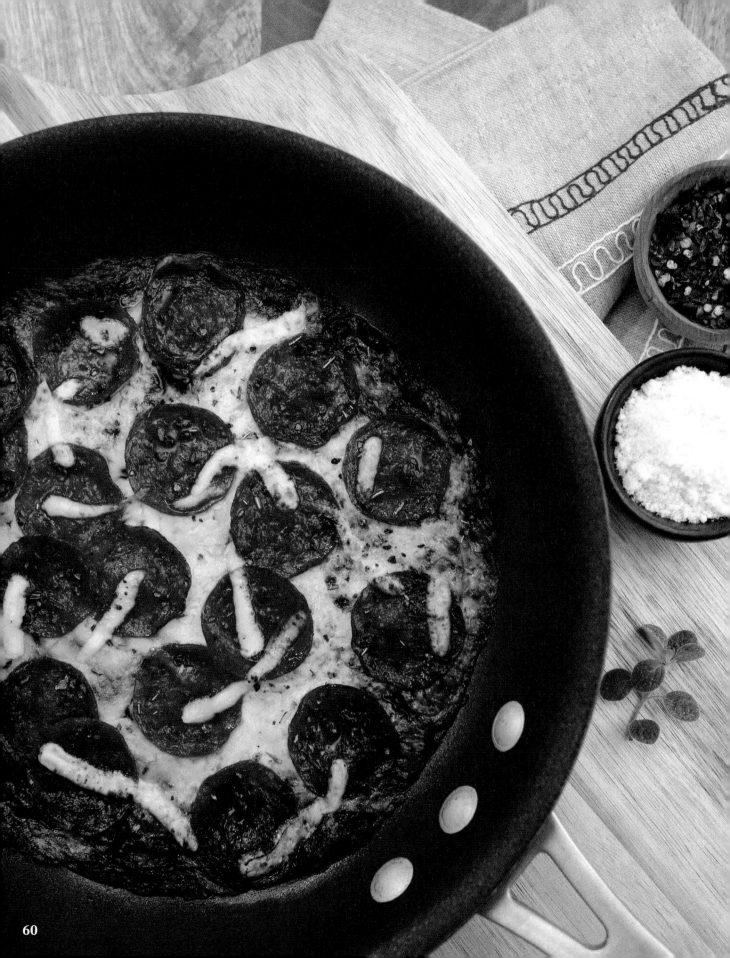

SKILLET PIZZA

FIVE MINUTE PEPPERONI PERFECTION

This is one of those easily thrown together recipes that I've cooked too many times to count. With a crust made of mozzarella cheese, there's no knead to go kneading dough to have the great flavors of pizza any time!

SHOPPING LIST

1¼ cups shredded mozzarella cheese, divided

¼ teaspoon dried oregano

⅛ teaspoon garlic powder

⅛ teaspoon salt

2 ounces sliced pepperoni

HELPFUL TIPS

This is how I've always made this, without sauce, but you can always add a thin layer of pizza sauce (without added sugar) over the crust before adding the top layer of cheese.

1 PLACE a 10-inch oven-safe nonstick skillet over medium heat.

2 FILL the bottom of the pan with ¾ cup of mozzarella cheese, leaving about an inch of surface around the cheese as room to flip with a spatula.

3 SPRINKLE the cheese with oregano, garlic powder, and salt.

4 LET cook for 3 minutes, without touching, or until the bottom of the cheese is golden brown.

5 SLIDE a spatula under the cheese and flip. You now have a cheesy crust!

6 TOP the crust with the remaining ½ cup of mozzarella cheese, and the sliced pepperoni.

7 SET the broiler to high, and place the skillet under the broiler for 2 minutes, just until pepperoni has crisped up. For best texture, let cool for 3 minutes before cutting into wedges to serve.

WHAT MAKES IT QUICK & EASY: This is just about the fastest pizza around!

Calories: 190 • Fat: 15.5g • Protein: 11.5g • Total Carbs: 0.5g – Fiber: 0g = **Net Carbs: 0.5g**

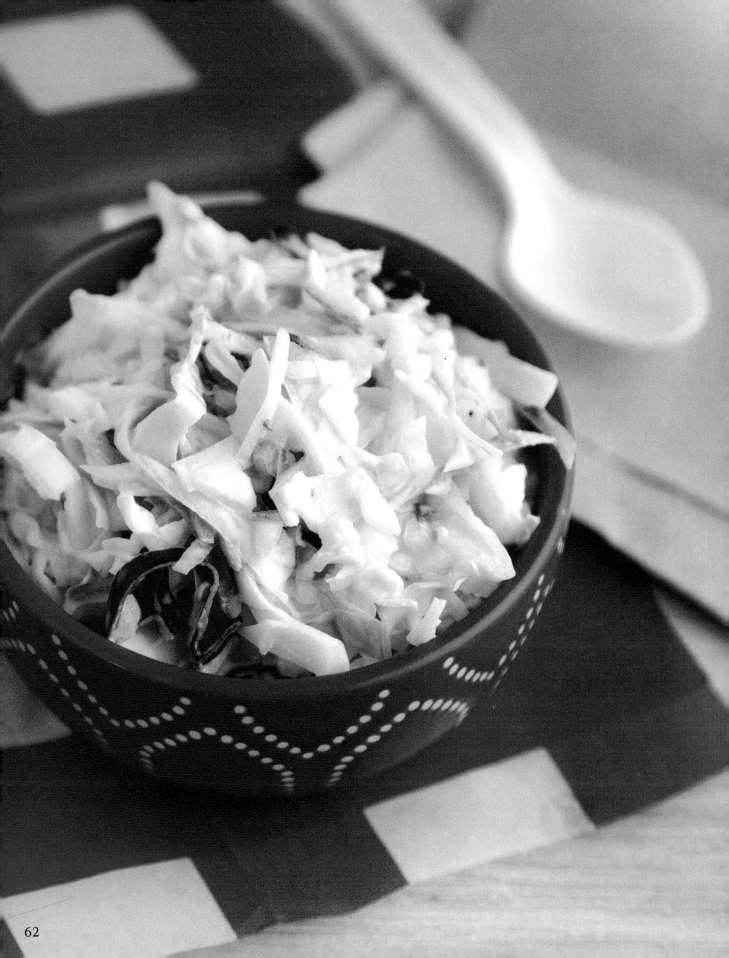

FAST FOOD COLESLAW

YOU'LL SWEAR YOU DROVE THROUGH KENTUCKY

Copycat "Kentucky-style" coleslaw recipes have been some of the most popular recipes online for years now. My take on this fast food staple's secret recipe cuts the sugar while also ditching finely shredded or grated cabbage for standard coleslaw mix that you can buy pre-shredded.

SHOPPING LIST

DRESSING

½ cup mayonnaise

½ cup half-and-half

¼ cup sugar substitute

2 tablespoons white vinegar

1 teaspoon lemon juice

½ teaspoon salt

½ teaspoon black pepper

SLAW

1 (16-ounce) bag shredded coleslaw cabbage mix

3 tablespoons minced yellow onion

1 ADD all Dressing ingredients to a large food storage container, and whisk to combine.

2 ADD the Slaw ingredients into the Dressing, folding until well coated.

3 FOR best flavor, cover and refrigerate for at least 2 hours before serving.

HELPFUL TIPS

Typical copycat recipes call for buttermilk, which is high in carbs. I replicate that flavor by using half-and-half and a small amount of lemon juice.

WHAT MAKES IT QUICK & EASY: Using pre-shredded coleslaw mix cuts the most intensive prep-work out of making coleslaw.

Calories: 175 • Fat: 16g • Protein: 2g • Total Carbs: 7g − Fiber: 1.5g = **Net Carbs: 5.5g**

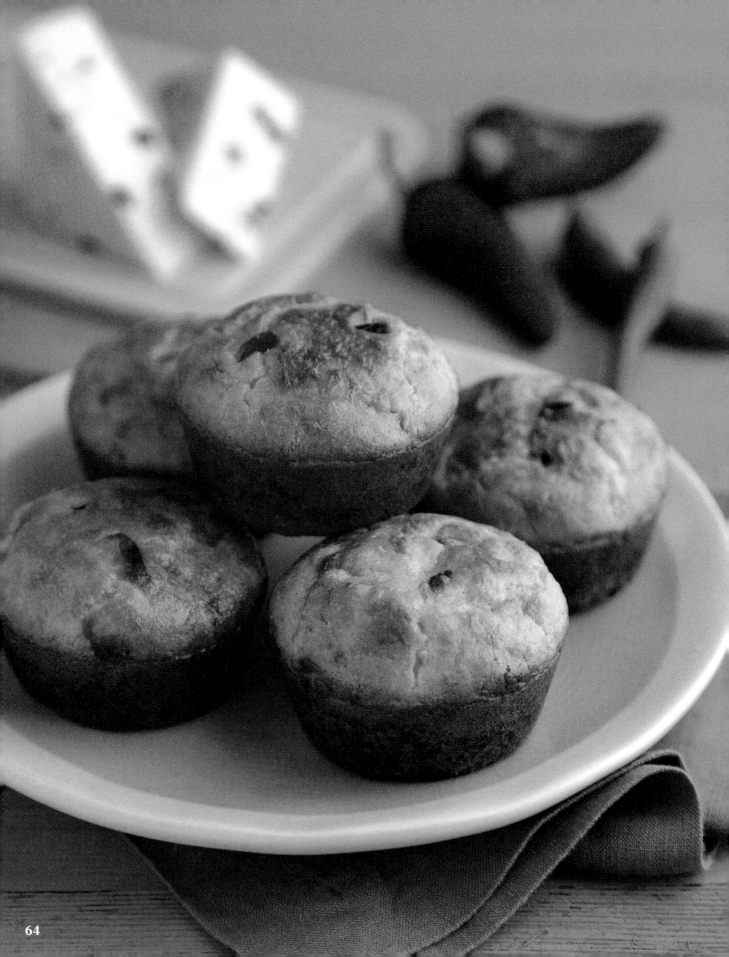

PEPPER JACK "CORN" MUFFINS

A PERFECT LUNCH-TIME SIDE

These savory muffins with a hint of sweetness are actually made without any corn at all, but you don't have to tell anyone that! Pepper jack cheese adds a bit of heat that goes great with the corn flavors created through the use of butter extract and a touch of vanilla extract. Serve alongside salads or soups for a full lunch.

LUNCH

SHOPPING LIST

Nonstick cooking spray

1 cup blanched almond flour

¼ cup sugar substitute

1½ teaspoons baking powder

2 large eggs

¼ cup heavy cream

½ teaspoon butter extract

¼ teaspoon vanilla extract

½ cup shredded pepper jack cheese

HELPFUL TIPS

An ice cream scoop is the perfect size for filling the muffin cups with the batter in this recipe.

1 PLACE oven rack in the center position and preheat to 375°F. Spray a 6-cup muffin pan with nonstick cooking spray.

2 IN a mixing bowl, combine the almond flour, sugar substitute, and baking powder.

3 IN a separate mixing bowl, whisk together the eggs, heavy cream, butter extract, and vanilla extract.

4 FOLD the wet ingredients into the dry ingredients, then fold the pepper jack cheese into the batter, until all is combined.

5 SPOON the batter equally between the 6 greased muffin cups.

6 BAKE for 20 minutes, or until lightly browned, and a toothpick inserted into the center of a muffin comes out mostly clean. Serve warm.

WHAT MAKES IT QUICK & EASY: Other than the cheese, all of these ingredients are staples of any low-carb pantry.

Calories: 190 • Fat: 16g • Protein: 8.5g • Total Carbs: 6g – Fiber: 2g = **Net Carbs: 4g**

ZUCCHINI & ONION SALAD

MARINATED WITH VINEGAR AND FRESH OREGANO

This twist on a marinated cucumber and onion salad uses zucchini in place of the cucumbers and red onion in place of yellow or white onion. To go with the more Mediterranean vegetables, I like to use oregano to freshen things up.

SHOPPING LIST

2 large zucchini, thinly sliced

½ red onion, thinly sliced

¼ cup cider vinegar

2 tablespoons water

2 tablespoons sugar substitute

1 tablespoon chopped fresh oregano

½ teaspoon salt

¼ teaspoon black pepper

1 IN a food storage container, combine all ingredients, tossing to mix.

2 COVER and refrigerate for at least 2 hours before serving.

HELPFUL TIPS

Make this into a creamy salad by stirring in ⅓ cup of sour cream just before serving (after chilling for 2 hours).

WHAT MAKES IT QUICK & EASY: This salad is quickly pickled and ready to eat in only 2 hours, though it is even better after 6 hours.

Calories: 40 • Fat: 0g • Protein: 2g • Total Carbs: 7.5g − Fiber: 2g = **Net Carbs: 5.5g**

LUNCH

AVOCADO & MELON SALAD

WITH TOMATO, BASIL, AND BALSAMIC VINEGAR

Creamy avocado goes amazingly well with sweet cantaloupe and acidic tomato in this quick picnic salad. It's a perfectly refreshing taste of summer that you should serve ice cold.

SHOPPING LIST

2 cups chopped cantaloupe melon

1 Hass avocado, pitted, peeled, and chopped

1 tomato, chopped

2 tablespoons extra-virgin olive oil

2 tablespoons chopped fresh basil

¼ teaspoon salt

¼ teaspoon black pepper

2 teaspoons balsamic vinegar

1 IN a mixing bowl, toss together all ingredients, except balsamic vinegar.

2 DRIZZLE balsamic vinegar over salad before serving.

HELPFUL TIPS

Honeydew melon, or a combination of honeydew and cantaloupe can be used as the melon in this recipe.

WHAT MAKES IT QUICK & EASY: We make this much quicker by buying pre-cut cantaloupe.

Calories: 155 • Fat: 13g • Protein: 2g • Total Carbs: 10.5g – Fiber: 2.5g = **Net Carbs: 8g**

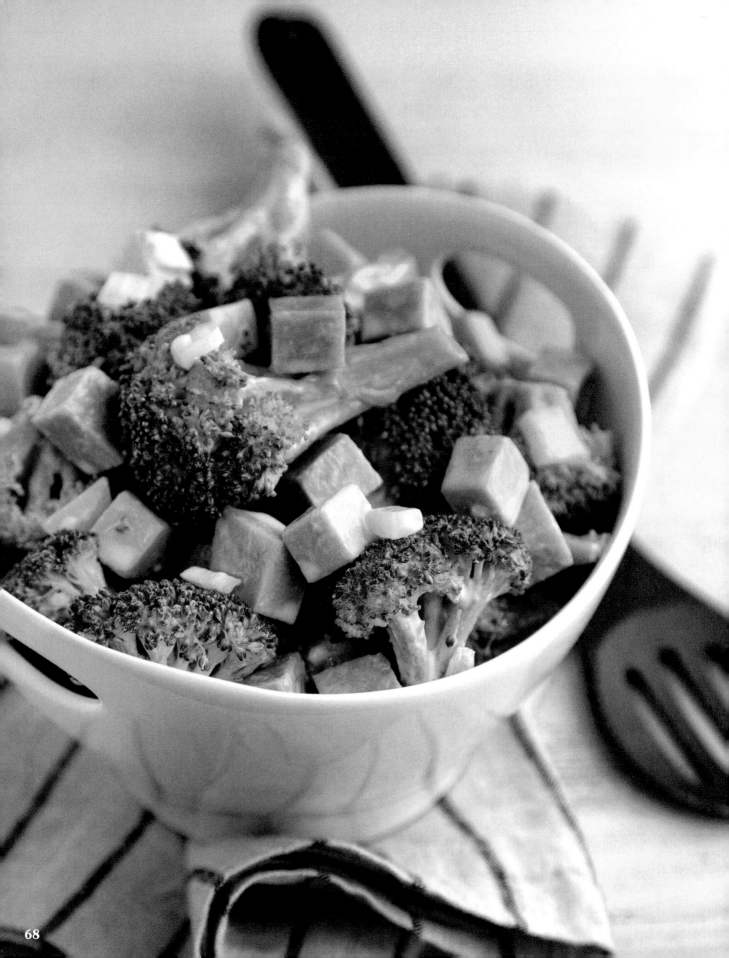

THE BEST BROCCOLI SALAD
WITH ONION, CHEDDAR, AND HAM

This is the perfect potluck salad, as it is sure to please just about anyone that passes by! You can't ever go wrong with the classic combination of broccoli, ham, and cheese—and especially not when you toss it in a simple, coleslaw-style dressing like the dressing in this recipe.

SHOPPING LIST

1 pound fresh broccoli florets

2 tablespoons cider vinegar

½ teaspoon salt

4 ounces cubed ham

4 ounces sharp Cheddar cheese, cubed

3 tablespoons diced yellow onion

¼ cup sour cream

¼ cup half-and-half

2 tablespoons mayonnaise

1 tablespoon sugar substitute

¼ teaspoon black pepper

1 IN a large food storage container, toss together broccoli florets, cider vinegar, and salt. For best texture, cover and refrigerate at least 1 hour before continuing.

2 ONCE broccoli has marinated in the vinegar, add all remaining ingredients and toss to combine.

3 FOR best flavor, cover and refrigerate at least 2 additional hours before serving.

HELPFUL TIPS

Marinating the broccoli in only the vinegar and salt will help soften the broccoli before adding the sour cream and mayonnaise, which will cut the acidity of the vinegar.

WHAT MAKES IT QUICK & EASY: Using a bag of pre-cut broccoli florets and using pre-cubed ham makes this recipe much lighter on prep than it first looks.

Calories: 190 • Fat: 13.5g • Protein: 10.5g • Total Carbs: 7g – Fiber: 2g = **Net Carbs: 5g**

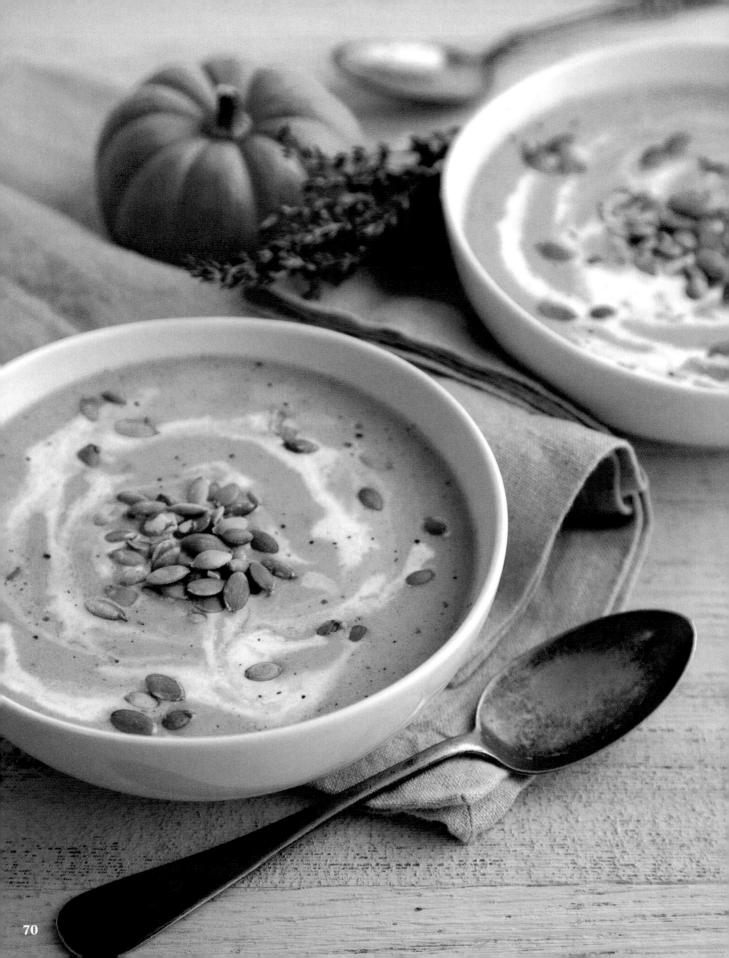

PREP TIME: 10 MIN • COOK TIME: 13 MIN • SERVES: 4

PUMPKIN SOUP

TOPPED WITH SHELLED PUMPKIN SEEDS

This velvety rich soup is both sweet and savory, with just a touch of fall spices to warm your senses. While the soup has heavy cream mixed in, I like to drizzle just a little bit extra into each bowl, just before serving, to get the results seen in the picture at left.

LUNCH

SHOPPING LIST

2 tablespoons unsalted butter
½ cup diced yellow onion
2¼ cups water
1 (15-ounce) can pure pumpkin
⅓ cup heavy cream
¼ cup sugar substitute
1 tablespoon chicken base
1½ teaspoons dry rubbed sage
¼ teaspoon dried thyme
¼ teaspoon allspice
¼ teaspoon salt
¼ cup roasted pepitas (shelled pumpkin seeds)

1. Heat butter in a large sauce pot over medium-high heat, until sizzling.
2. Place yellow onion in the hot pot and sauté 3 minutes.
3. Add all remaining ingredients, except pepitas, to the pot and stir to combine.
4. Stirring frequently, bring the soup up to a simmer.
5. Reduce heat to medium and, stirring frequently, let simmer 10 minutes.
6. Remove from heat and let rest 1 minute before serving topped with the roasted pepitas.

HELPFUL TIPS

You can usually find the shelled and roasted pumpkin seeds (often labeled as "pepitas") with other gourmet seeds and nuts in the produce section of the grocery store.

WHAT MAKES IT QUICK & EASY: Using canned pumpkin makes this into a recipe that you can make all year round, and without the Hassle of carving a whole pumpkin!

Calories: 185 • Fat: 13.5g • Protein: 3.5g • Total Carbs: 12.5g – Fiber: 3.5g = **Net Carbs: 9g**

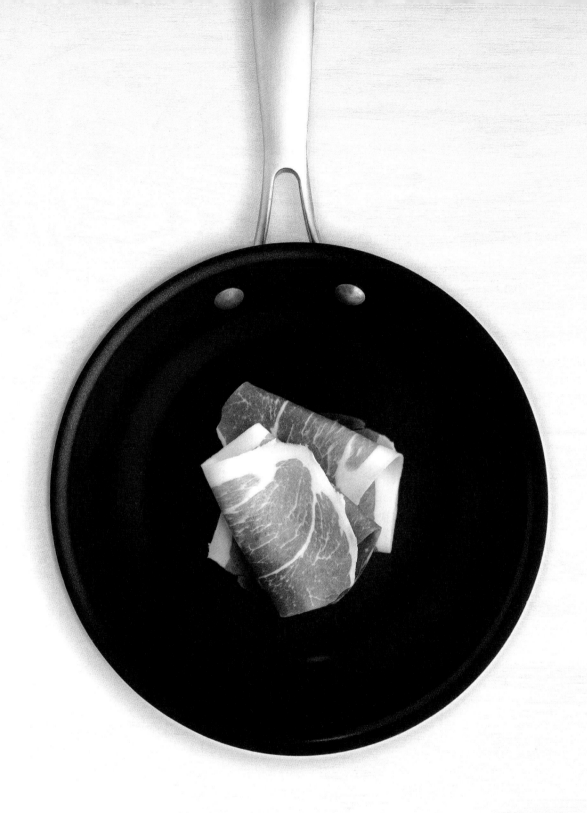

APPETIZERS & SNACKS

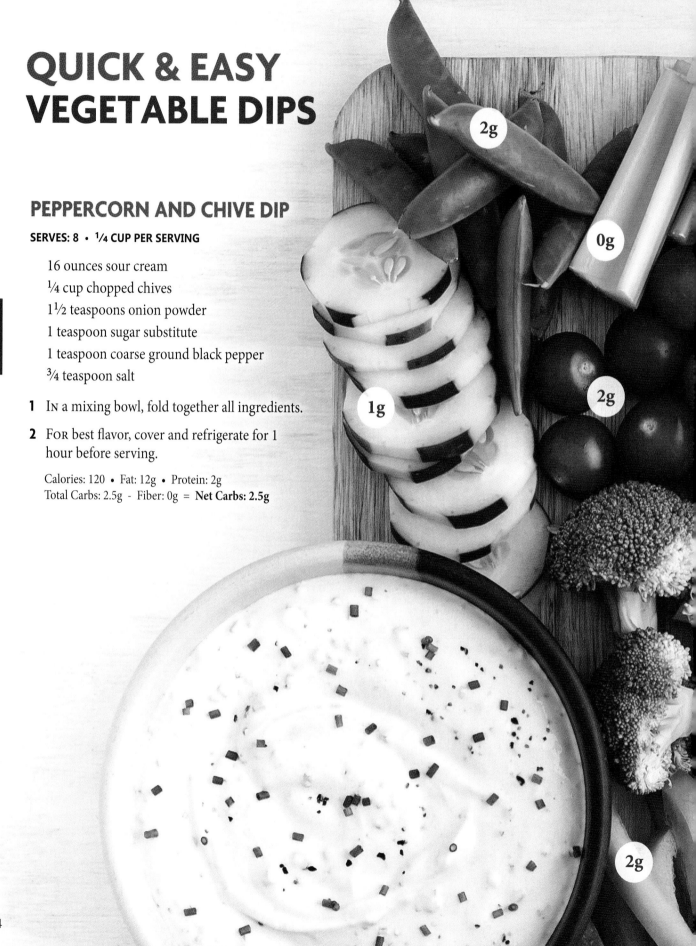

QUICK & EASY VEGETABLE DIPS

PEPPERCORN AND CHIVE DIP

SERVES: 8 • ¼ CUP PER SERVING

16 ounces sour cream
¼ cup chopped chives
1½ teaspoons onion powder
1 teaspoon sugar substitute
1 teaspoon coarse ground black pepper
¾ teaspoon salt

1 IN a mixing bowl, fold together all ingredients.

2 FOR best flavor, cover and refrigerate for 1 hour before serving.

Calories: 120 • Fat: 12g • Protein: 2g
Total Carbs: 2.5g - Fiber: 0g = **Net Carbs: 2.5g**

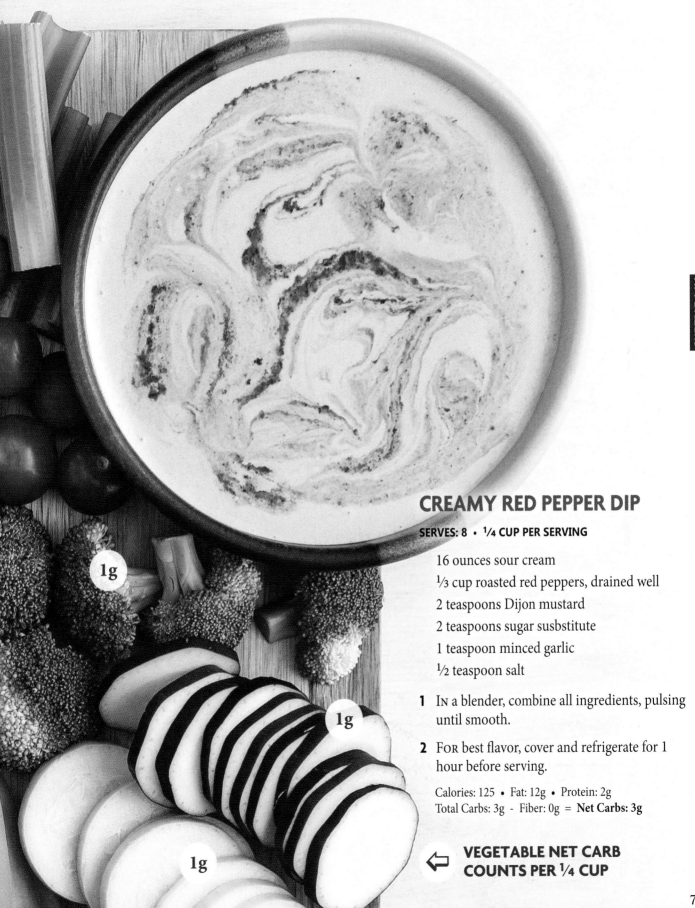

1g

1g

1g

CREAMY RED PEPPER DIP

SERVES: 8 • ¼ CUP PER SERVING

16 ounces sour cream

⅓ cup roasted red peppers, drained well

2 teaspoons Dijon mustard

2 teaspoons sugar susbstitute

1 teaspoon minced garlic

½ teaspoon salt

1 IN a blender, combine all ingredients, pulsing until smooth.

2 FOR best flavor, cover and refrigerate for 1 hour before serving.

Calories: 125 • Fat: 12g • Protein: 2g
Total Carbs: 3g - Fiber: 0g = **Net Carbs: 3g**

⬅ **VEGETABLE NET CARB COUNTS PER ¼ CUP**

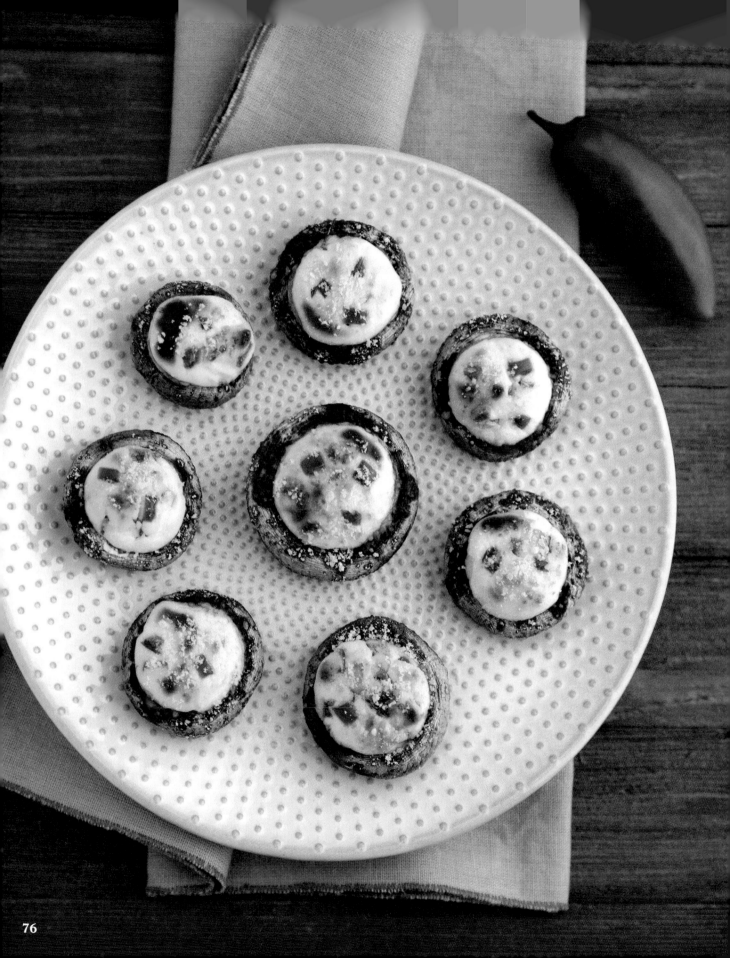

JALAPEÑO POPPER STUFFED MUSHROOMS

ONCE YOU POP, IT'S HARD TO STOP

I love to combine comfort foods to create something entirely new. In this recipe, I've combined two classic appetizers—stuffed mushrooms and jalapeño poppers—into a perfect palate pleaser for any party.

SHOPPING LIST

Nonstick cooking spray

1 pound large button mushrooms (about 16 mushrooms)

Salt, to season

4 ounces cream cheese, softened

2 jalapeños, seeded and finely diced

1 large egg white

¼ teaspoon salt

1 tablespoon grated Parmesan cheese

HELPFUL TIPS

For even more browning, you can place these under the broiler for 2 minutes after baking.

1 PREHEAT oven to 375°F. Spray a sheet pan with nonstick cooking spray.

2 SCRUB mushrooms clean. Remove stems and discard. Sprinkle the insides of the mushrooms with salt to season.

3 PLACE cream cheese, jalapeños, egg white, and ¼ teaspoon of salt in a mixing bowl, and whisk with a fork until well combined.

4 STUFF each mushroom until overflowing with the filling.

5 PLACE the stuffed mushrooms on the prepared sheet pan. Sprinkle Parmesan cheese over top of all.

6 BAKE for 15 minutes, or until mushrooms are tender and filling is beginning to rise out of the mushrooms.

WHAT MAKES IT QUICK & EASY: Making traditional jalapeño poppers requires breading soft cream cheese, freezing, deep frying, and hoping they don't explode!

Calories: 135 · Fat: 10.5g · Protein: 7.5g · Total Carbs: 4.5g − Fiber: 1.5g = **Net Carbs: 3g**

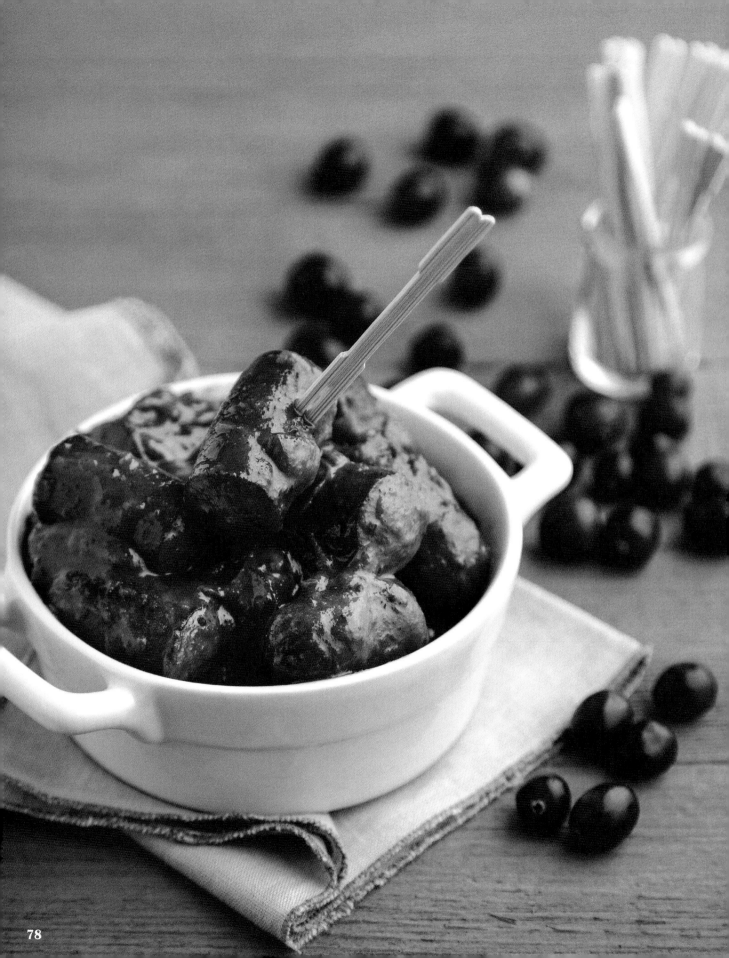

CRANBERRY COCKTAIL FRANKS

MADE WITH FRESH CRANBERRIES AND ALL-NATURAL HOT DOGS

Cocktail franks like these are a potluck staple that is often made with either canned cranberry sauce or grape jelly. Both are full of sugar or corn syrup, so I've made my version using real, fresh cranberries, cooked from scratch. I've also avoided using true cocktail-sized smoked sausages, as those have corn syrup and nitrates added!

SHOPPING LIST

2 teaspoons vegetable oil

8 all-natural hot dogs, cut into thirds

¼ cup diced yellow onion

8 ounces fresh cranberries

¾ cup water

¾ cup sugar substitute

1 tablespoon Dijon mustard

¼ teaspoon onion powder

Baking soda (see tip)

HELPFUL TIPS

Adding baking soda can cut the tart acidity of the cranberries. If the sauce is too tart for your liking, stir ¼ teaspoon of baking soda at a time into the pot, until it is at your liking. The sauce will bubble up green, but don't worry, that is just the baking soda neutralizing the acid of the berries. It will dissipate as you stir it in. I found that ¾ teaspoon of baking soda makes for a nice, mellow sauce.

1 HEAT vegetable oil in a large sauce pot over medium-high heat, until hot.

2 PLACE cut hot dogs in the pot and brown.

3 ADD the yellow onion to the pot and sauté for 2 minutes, just until onions sweat.

4 ADD the cranberries, water, sugar substitute, Dijon, and onion powder to the pot, and stir to combine.

5 BRING up to a simmer, reduce heat to medium, and let simmer, stirring occasionally, for 15 minutes. Cranberries should have cooked down, into a sauce.

6 REMOVE from heat, and add baking soda to taste to reduce acidity (see tip). Let rest 5 minutes to further thicken before serving.

APPETIZERS

WHAT MAKES IT QUICK & EASY: Even though this is entirely made from scratch, it is still made in only minutes, whereas traditional versions take hours in a slow cooker.

Calories: 150 · Fat: 9.5g · Protein: 7g · Total Carbs: 5.5g − Fiber: 1g = **Net Carbs: 4.5g**

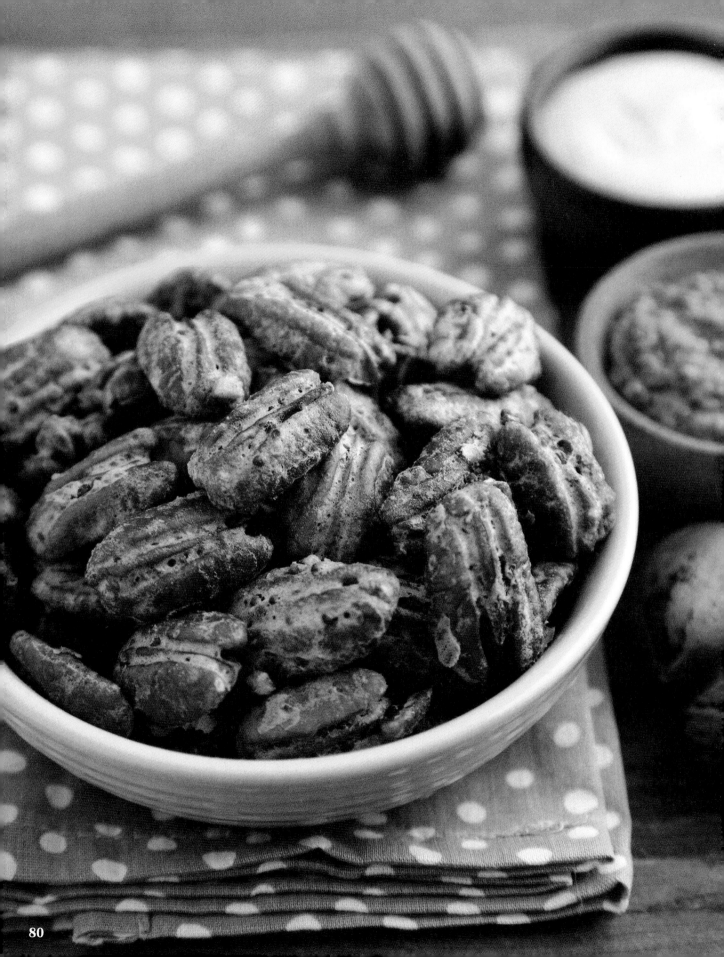

HONEY MUSTARD PECANS

SWEET AND SALTY SNACKING MADE EASY

I always like to keep the pantry stocked with different nuts and seeds for baking dessert recipes—but more importantly—general snacking! When I get tired of plain roasted nuts, I go to the drawing board to come up with new flavors. Even I was surprised by how much mustard flavor I could bake into these sweet pecans, without the need for the flavored powders that snack food manufacturers use.

SHOPPING LIST

1 large egg white, beaten

3 tablespoons sugar substitute

2 tablespoons yellow mustard

1 tablespoon coarse deli mustard

8 ounces shelled pecan halves

HELPFUL TIPS

You can simply use an extra tablespoon of the yellow mustard in place of the coarse deli mustard, to simplify your shopping list.

1 PREHEAT oven to 300°F. Line a sheet pan with parchment paper.

2 IN a large mixing bowl, whisk together egg white, sugar substitute, yellow mustard, and deli mustard.

3 ADD the pecans to the mustard mixture, and toss to fully coat all.

4 SPREAD the coated pecans out onto the prepared sheet pan.

5 BAKE for 20 minutes, flipping halfway through. Let cool for 5 minutes before serving.

WHAT MAKES IT QUICK & EASY: Having snacks like these on hand makes it easier to stick to your low-carb goals!

Calories: 205 • Fat: 20.5g • Protein: 4g • Total Carbs: 5g – Fiber: 3g = **Net Carbs: 2g**

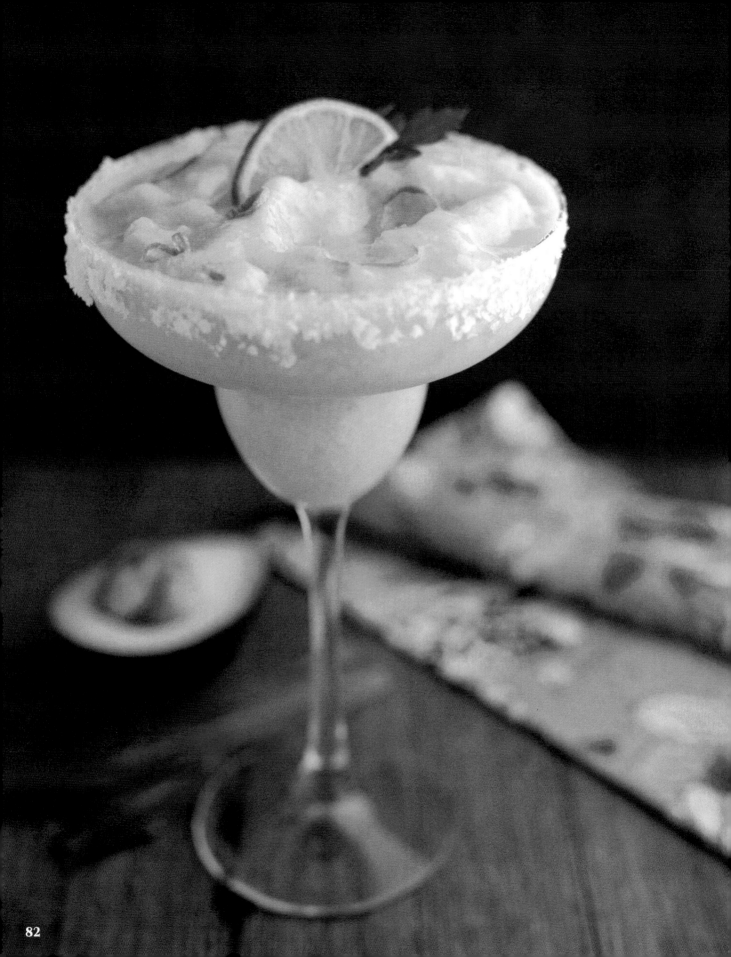

AVOCADO MARGARITAS
WITH OR WITHOUT TEQUILA

Adding avocado to these refreshing margaritas makes for an extra-creamy drink that tastes far better than you may think. The avocado tastes more like melon once it has been sweetened, but it's the smooth texture that steals the show. Nutritional information is for the drink when made with tequila.

SHOPPING LIST

2 cups Fresca grapefruit soda

2 cups ice

½ medium avocado, peeled and pitted

2 ounces tequila, optional (see tip)

2 tablespoons lime juice

2 tablespoons sugar substitute

Lime slices, for glass rim

Coarse margarita-salt, for glass rim

Orange zest, for garnish

HELPFUL TIPS

I like to use silver tequila in this, however this is also absolutely delicious when made "virgin" with no alcohol at all.

1 ADD Fresca, ice, avocado, tequila (if using), lime juice, and sugar substitute to a blender.

2 BLEND 2 minutes, until completely smooth.

3 MEANWHILE, rub the rims of 2 large margarita glasses with a slice of lime to wet them.

4 DIP the rims of the glasses into the coarse salt to coat.

5 POUR the blended margarita into the glasses and garnish with orange zest, if desired.

APPETIZERS

WHAT MAKES IT QUICK & EASY: This one-blender treat is easily whipped up in less than 5 minutes.

Calories: 145 • Fat: 6g • Protein: 1.5g • Total Carbs: 5.5g − Fiber: 1.5g = **Net Carbs: 4g**

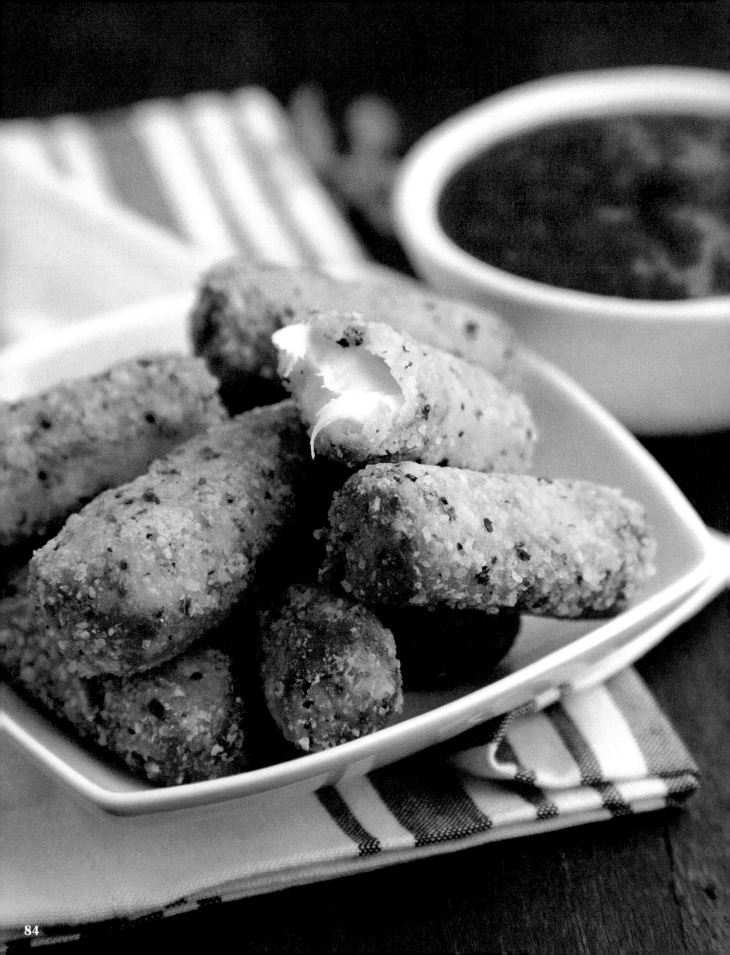

MOZZARELLA STICKS

BREADED WITHOUT ANY BREAD AT ALL

Your party guests will never believe that these mozzarella sticks are not just low-carb, but breaded without any type of flour whatsoever. Double-breading the mozzarella in grated Parmesan cheese makes a thick shell that looks, tastes, and has all the crunch of ordinary mozzarella sticks.

SHOPPING LIST

6 mozzarella string cheese sticks

2 large eggs

⅔ cup grated Parmesan cheese

1 teaspoon Italian seasoning

¼ teaspoon black pepper

Vegetable oil, for shallow frying

Pasta sauce, for dipping, optional

HELPFUL TIPS

Freezing the mozzarella sticks before frying ensures that the cheese melts just as the breading is fully browned, and doesn't escape any earlier.

1 CUT each mozzarella stick into 2 shorter sticks.

2 IN a shallow but wide bowl, whisk eggs to create an egg wash.

3 IN a separate bowl, combine Parmesan cheese, Italian seasoning, and pepper to create a breading.

4 DIP each cut piece of mozzarella in the egg wash, flipping to thoroughly coat. Transfer to the breading mixture, and press into the cheese to ensure the breading adheres.

5 DOUBLE-BREAD each stick by going back into the egg wash and then back into Parmesan for a second coat, ensuring that each cheese stick is fully breaded.

6 COVER and place breaded cheese sticks in the freezer for at least 1 hour before preparing.

7 FILL a large skillet with about ¾-inch of vegetable oil and place over medium-high heat. Let the oil heat up for about 2 minutes.

8 PLACE the frozen cheese sticks in the skillet, and cook until golden brown, about 5 minutes, flipping halfway through. Do this in two batches if your skillet is too small.

9 TRANSFER mozzarella sticks to paper towels to drain before serving alongside pasta sauce, for dipping, if desired.

WHAT MAKES IT QUICK & EASY: While I can't claim that these are as easy to make as store-bought sticks, I can guarantee that they are FAR lower in carbs!

Calories: 215 · Fat: 18g · Protein: 13.5g · Total Carbs: 1g – Fiber: 0g = **Net Carbs: 1g**

APPETIZERS

TURKEY-WRAPPED ASPARAGUS
WITH SMOKED PROVOLONE CHEESE

These little roll-ups make the perfect party alternative to pinwheels wrapped in high-carb flour tortillas. With the turkey and cheese on the outside, you put a crisp stalk of asparagus on the inside for flavor, texture, and stability of the wraps.

SHOPPING LIST

16 large asparagus tips

8 large slices deli turkey breast (rectangle or oval)

8 slices smoked provolone cheese

1/3 cup mayonnaise

HELPFUL TIPS

You can also do this with herbed cream cheese in place of the mayonnaise for even more flavor. Let it come to room temperature for easier spreading.

1 BOIL asparagus tips for 3 minutes, just until slightly tender, but still crisp. Drain and run under cold water.

2 CUT each slice of turkey in half cross-wise (across the shorter length), then cut each slice of provolone in half.

3 PLACE a half-slice of provolone over each of the half-slices of turkey.

4 SPREAD about 1 teaspoon of mayonnaise over each turkey and cheese stack.

5 PLACE a cooked asparagus tip over the top of the mayonnaise, then roll the turkey and cheese up and around the asparagus, eventually wrapping it around itself. Place each wrap on a serving platter, seam-side down, to better hold together. Serve immediately.

WHAT MAKES IT QUICK & EASY: These only look like they took a lot of work to make.

Calories: 190 • Fat: 14g • Protein: 12g • Total Carbs: 3g – Fiber: 1g = **Net Carbs: 2g**

APPETIZERS

JALAPEÑO SKINS

FILLED WITH CHEDDAR, BACON, AND SOUR CREAM

These spicy little bites are a new take on potato skins, with hollowed out jalapeño peppers in place of the potato skins themselves. All of the other classic flavors are still there though, so you'll be sure to get your fill of bacon, sour cream, chives, and melted Cheddar cheese— you're just getting those flavors in a new way.

SHOPPING LIST

Nonstick cooking spray

8 large jalapeño peppers

1 cup shredded sharp Cheddar cheese

¼ cup crumbled cooked bacon

¼ cup sour cream

2 tablespoons chopped chives

HELPFUL TIPS

Precooked and crumbled "bacon pieces" can be purchased in the salad dressing aisle to make this without having to cook or crumble your own bacon.

1 SPRAY a sheet pan with nonstick cooking spray.

2 CUT jalapeño peppers in half length-wise, and scoop out all seeds, discarding seeds.

3 LAY the halved peppers out on the prepared sheet pan, and fill each pepper with 1 tablespoon of the shredded Cheddar cheese. Sprinkle the crumbled bacon over the top of all.

4 PLACE oven rack two positions from the top of the oven, and set the broiler to high.

5 BROIL peppers for 3 minutes, or until cheese is bubbly hot, and just starting to brown.

6 TOP each pepper with a small dollop of sour cream, and sprinkle with chopped chives before serving.

APPETIZERS

WHAT MAKES IT QUICK & EASY: Making traditional potato skins requires boiling potatoes, scooping out the potato, then deep frying the skins before you can broil!

Calories: 105 • Fat: 8.5g • Protein: 5.5g • Total Carbs: 2.5g – Fiber: 1g = **Net Carbs: 1.5g**

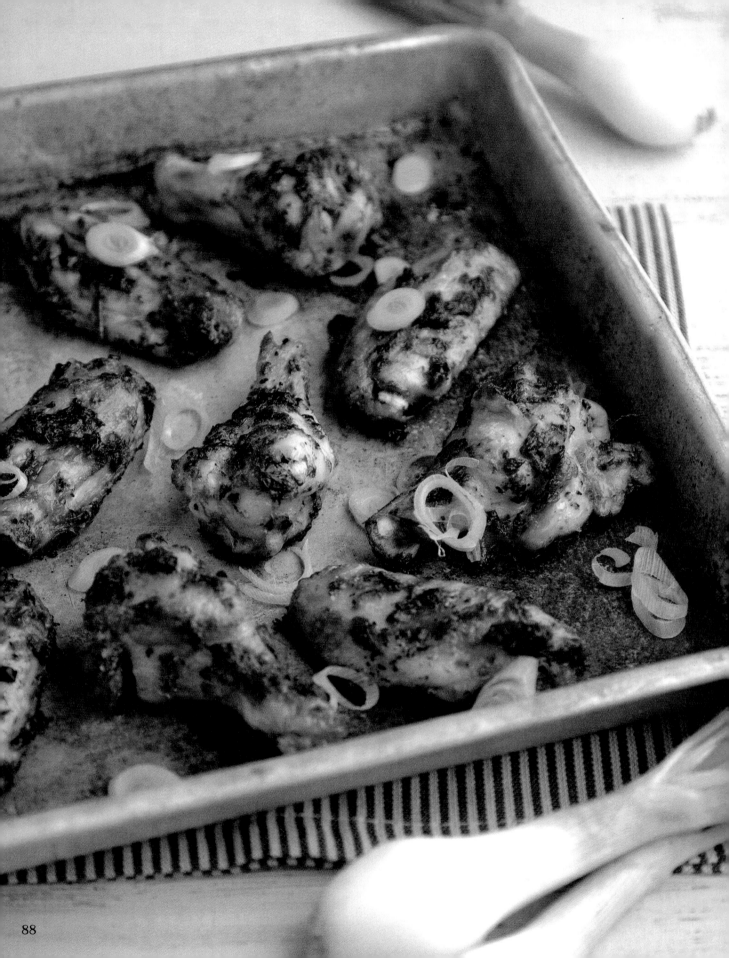

SWEET ONION CHICKEN WINGS
AN ADDICTIVE PARTY APPETIZER

Before baking, these chicken wings are tossed in a purée of green onions and olive oil, similar to pesto, but with an entirely different flavor. While the onion may seem overwhelming at first, it mellows out as the chicken wings bake, ending up very sweet and mild.

SHOPPING LIST

3 pounds fresh chicken wings, drum and wing separated

1 small bunch green onions

3 tablespoons olive oil

2 teaspoons sugar substitute

1 teaspoon white wine vinegar

½ teaspoon onion powder

½ teaspoon salt

½ teaspoon black pepper

HELPFUL TIPS

For a bit of heat, you can add 1 seeded jalapeño to the marinade before blending.

APPETIZERS

1 PREHEAT oven to 375°F. Line a sheet pan with aluminum foil.

2 PLACE chicken wings in a large mixing bowl.

3 IN a food processor, blend all remaining ingredients into a thick marinade.

4 ADD the blended onion marinade to the chicken wings and toss to fully coat each wing.

5 SPREAD the wings out onto the prepared sheet pan, arranging in a single layer.

6 BAKE for 50–55 minutes, or until slicing into the thickest drum reveals no pink. Serve immediately.

WHAT MAKES IT QUICK & EASY: By blending the marinade, there is no need to chop any ingredients.

Calories: 350 • Fat: 27.5g • Protein: 25.5g • Total Carbs: 1g − Fiber: 0g = **Net Carbs: 1g**

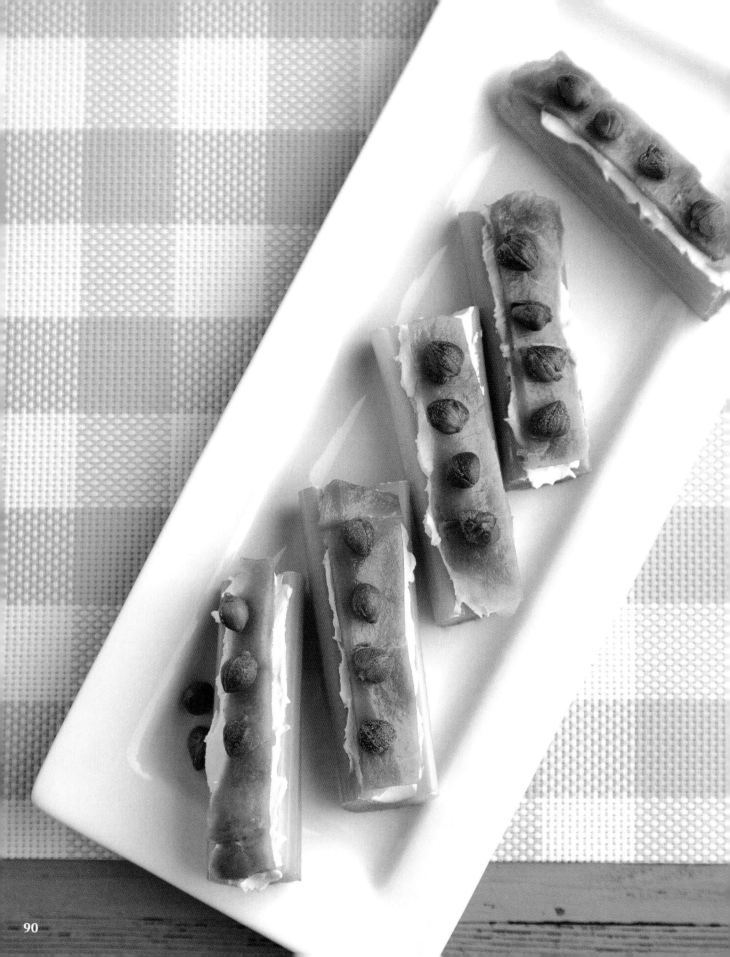

LOX ON A LOG

CELERY WITH CREAM CHEESE, SMOKED SALMON, AND CAPERS

This savory and playful twist on "Ants On a Log" reimagines that classic finger food for adults, with the tried and true flavors of smoked salmon and cream cheese. The "ants" in this case are capers in place of raisins, as capers are traditionally served over bagels with cream cheese and lox.

SHOPPING LIST

4 stalks celery, cut into thirds

4 ounces cream cheese, softened

2 ounces smoked salmon, sliced into strips

2 tablespoons capers, drained

APPETIZERS

1 SPREAD cream cheese into each piece of celery, until overflowing.

2 TOP the cream cheese on each piece of celery with a strip of smoked salmon.

3 ARRANGE capers over top of salmon before serving.

HELPFUL TIPS

While this looks best as pictured, it is easier and most practical to stick the capers into the cream cheese before topping with the salmon last— that way the capers do not roll off as you pick these up.

WHAT MAKES IT QUICK & EASY: With only a few ingredients and no cooking, this is a great appetizer to make when your oven or stove is tied up cooking dinner.

Calories: 80 • Fat: 7g • Protein: 3.5g • Total Carbs: 1g – Fiber: 0g = **Net Carbs: 1g**

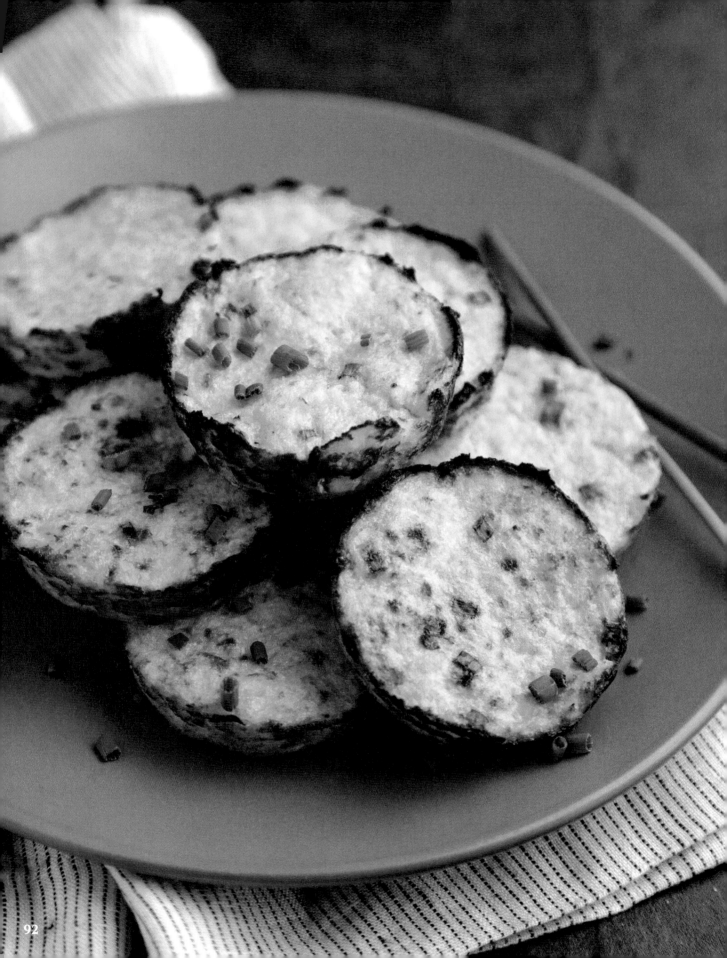

CHEESY CAULIFLOWER CROWNS
EXTRA-LARGE CAULIFLOWER TOTS WITH CHEDDAR

These large Cauliflower Crowns have the consistency and taste of tater tots, without the potato. Cheddar and Parmesan cheeses not only help to bind them together in place of breadcrumbs or potato starch, but adds extra cheesy goodness for a flavor you can't resist.

SHOPPING LIST

Nonstick cooking spray

1 (16-ounce) steam bag fresh cauliflower florets

⅔ cup shredded sharp Cheddar cheese

¼ cup grated Parmesan cheese

1 large egg

½ teaspoon onion powder

½ teaspoon salt

2 tablespoons chopped chives

HELPFUL TIPS

These will get soggy after being left out, and especially after refrigerating.
To crisp back up, simply bake on a sheet pan for 10 minutes at 350°F.

APPETIZERS

1 PLACE oven rack in the center position and preheat to 350°F. Spray a 12-cup muffin pan with nonstick cooking spray.

2 POKE holes in the bag of cauliflower to vent, then microwave for 3 minutes. Place in the freezer to cool down as you measure out the rest of the ingredients.

3 ADD Cheddar cheese, Parmesan cheese, egg, onion powder, salt, and the cooled cauliflower florets to a blender.

4 PULSE until all ingredients are mixed, but cauliflower is still a finely minced consistency, like rice.

5 FOLD the chopped chives into the cauliflower batter.

6 USING rounded tablespoons or 1-ounce ice cream scoop, split the batter evenly between the 12 greased muffin cups.

7 BAKE for 30 minutes or until sides look very crispy.

8 SET the broiler to high and broil for 4–5 minutes, or until the tops are golden brown. Let cool for 5 minutes before serving.

WHAT MAKES IT QUICK & EASY: Tater tots are something few people have ever tried to make at home, but these are made easy, with no need to form them into shapes by hand.

Calories: 102 · Fat: 6.5g · Protein: 7.5g · Total Carbs: 4.5g − Fiber: 2g = **Net Carbs: 2.5g**

ANTIPASTO VEGETABLE SALAD

WITH ARTICHOKES, OLIVES, ZUCCHINI, TOMATOES, AND MOZZARELLA

I always make sure I have an antipasto salad or platter at every holiday or family get-together. A quick tossed antipasto salad like this one can really brighten up a party buffet, without the cleanup of putting out multiple bowls of different pickles or marinated vegetables.

SHOPPING LIST

8 ounces mini fresh mozzarella balls, drained

1 (6.5-ounce) jar quartered marinated artichoke hearts, drained

1 (6-ounce) can whole pitted black olives, drained

1 large zucchini, chopped

1 cup grape tomatoes

3 tablespoons chopped fresh basil

2 tablespoons extra-virgin olive oil

2 tablespoons balsamic vinegar

¼ teaspoon garlic powder

¼ teaspoon salt

¼ teaspoon black pepper

1 IN a serving bowl, combine all ingredients, tossing to fully mix.

2 FOR better flavor, refrigerate for 1 hour before serving.

HELPFUL TIPS

A marinated olive mix goes great in this in place of the black olives. You can also add chopped salami or sliced pepperoni for a non-vegetarian salad.

WHAT MAKES IT QUICK & EASY: The zucchini and basil are the only ingredients in this salad that require chopping.

Calories: 270 • Fat: 23g • Protein: 8.5g • Total Carbs: 7.5g – Fiber: 2g = **Net Carbs: 5.5g**

APPETIZERS

BACON-WRAPPED CHICKEN TENDERS
WITH FRESH SAGE LEAVES

Everything is better with bacon, and that's a motto that I'll repeat a few times throughout this cookbook! Rather than bread and deep fry chicken tenders to high-carb results, I've wrapped them in crispy bacon for both texture and flavor. A whole sage leaf cooked between the bacon and the chicken makes these not only look better, but taste better too.

SHOPPING LIST

8 chicken tenderloins (about 1 pound)

Salt and black pepper

Garlic powder

8 leaves sage

8 slices thin-cut bacon

Nonstick cooking spray

HELPFUL TIPS

My Honey Dijon Dressing, recipe page: 50, makes a perfect dipping sauce for these.

1 GENEROUSLY season chicken tenderloins with salt, pepper, and garlic powder.

2 PLACE a sage leaf over each seasoned tenderloin.

3 WRAP a slice of bacon around each tenderloin in a spiral, securing the sage leaf in the process. For best results, hold the bacon in place by skewering each wrapped tender with a toothpick.

4 SPRAY a large skillet with nonstick cooking spray and place over medium-high heat.

5 ADD wrapped tenders to the skillet, and cook until bacon is crisp, about 5 minutes on each side. Transfer to paper towels to soak up excess grease before serving.

APPETIZERS

WHAT MAKES IT QUICK & EASY: These look far more difficult to make than they truly are, so you can make a big impression with very little work.

Calories: 150 · Fat: 9g · Protein: 16g · Total Carbs: 0.5g − Fiber: 0g = **Net Carbs: 0.5g**

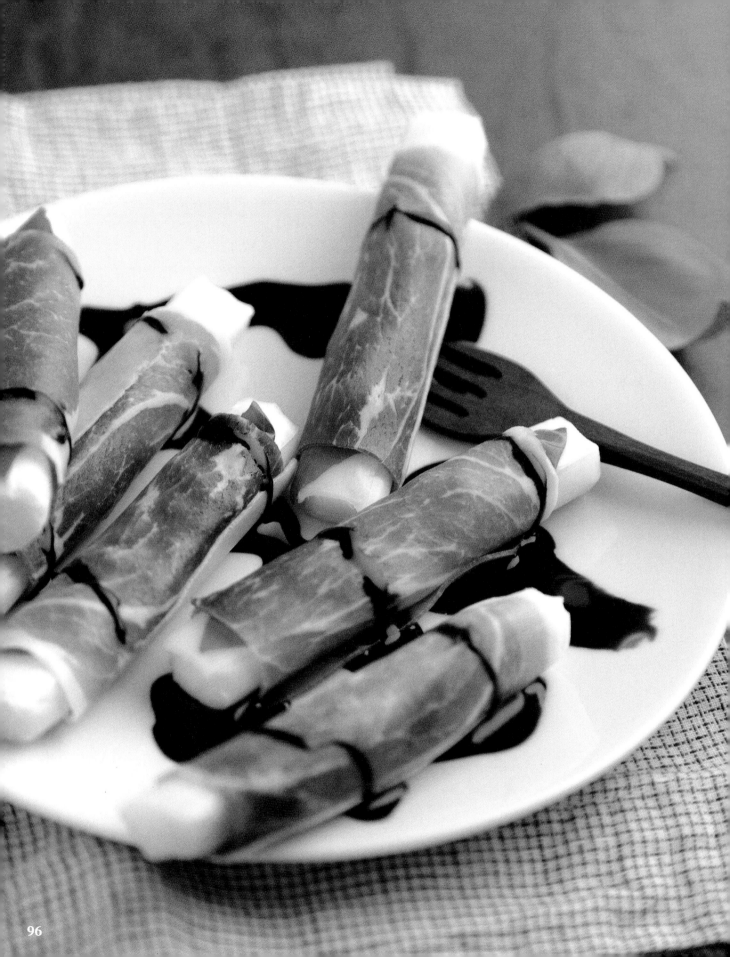

PROSCIUTTO PANINO ROLLS
WITH BASIL AND BALSAMIC VINEGAR

Panino rolls are one of my favorite appetizers, and we serve them at every single holiday. By making these prosciutto-wrapped mozzarella sticks fresh, I can make far more for the money than purchasing them pre-made. Plus, prosciutto purchased separately is almost always of a higher quality than the prosciutto used on store-bought paninos.

SHOPPING LIST

4 long slices prosciutto

16 leaves fresh basil

8 mozzarella string cheese sticks

1 tablespoon balsamic vinegar, if desired

HELPFUL TIPS

You can also do this with arugula in place of the basil for a peppery bite in place of the herbaceous flavor.

1 CUT each slice of prosciutto in half cross-wise (across the shorter length).

2 PLACE two leaves of basil over top of each of the 8 pieces of prosciutto.

3 PLACE a mozzarella stick over the top of the basil, then roll the prosciutto up and around the cheese, eventually wrapping it around itself. Place each panino on a serving platter, seam-side down to better hold together.

4 SERVE drizzled with balsamic vinegar, if desired.

APPETIZERS

WHAT MAKES IT QUICK & EASY: These can be rolled up in mere minutes, but make a big impact at parties.

Calories: 100 • Fat: 7g • Protein: 10g • Total Carbs: 1g – Fiber: 0g = **Net Carbs: 1g**

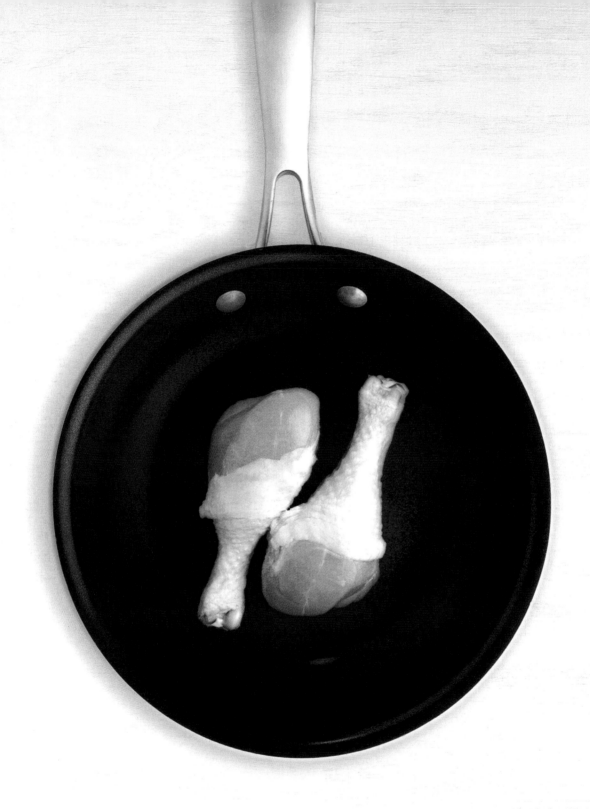

POULTRY

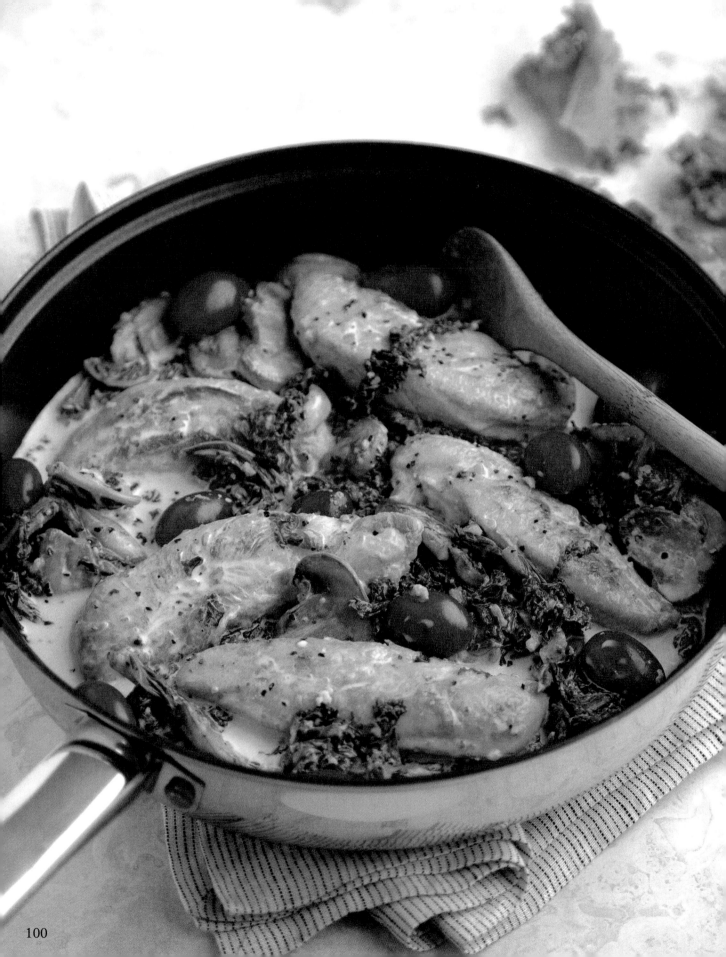

CREAMY CHICKEN & KALE SKILLET

WITH MUSHROOMS AND TOMATOES

Not only is this dish bursting with color, it's also bursting with fresh flavors! When you're cooking with color, you just know you're eating well. For a full meal, serve over one of my Pasta Alternatives, recipe page: 170.

SHOPPING LIST

1 tablespoon unsalted butter

2 teaspoons vegetable oil

1 pound chicken tenderloins

Salt and black pepper

8 ounces sliced mushrooms

1 teaspoon minced garlic

1 small bunch kale, chopped

¾ cup heavy cream

¼ cup grated Parmesan cheese

¾ cup grape tomatoes

HELPFUL TIPS

Pre-chopped kale can be purchased in large bags in the produce section to save on prep time.

1 HEAT butter and oil in a large skillet over medium-high heat, until sizzling.

2 GENEROUSLY season chicken tenderloins with salt and pepper.

3 PLACE seasoned tenderloins in the hot skillet, and brown well, about 4 minutes on each side. Remove from skillet and set aside.

4 PLACE the mushrooms and garlic in the empty skillet, and cook until mushrooms begin to brown.

5 ADD the kale to the skillet and cook, stirring frequently, until the kale is tender.

6 ADD the chicken tenderloins back into the skillet. Pour the heavy cream into the skillet and bring up to a simmer. Reduce heat to low and let simmer for 3 minutes.

7 REMOVE from heat and stir in Parmesan cheese and grape tomatoes. Season with salt and pepper to taste before serving.

POULTRY

WHAT MAKES IT QUICK & EASY: This is a great one-pot meal that cooks in only 15 minutes.

Calories: 310 · Fat: 16.5g · Protein: 33g · Total Carbs: 10g – Fiber: 2g = **Net Carbs: 8g**

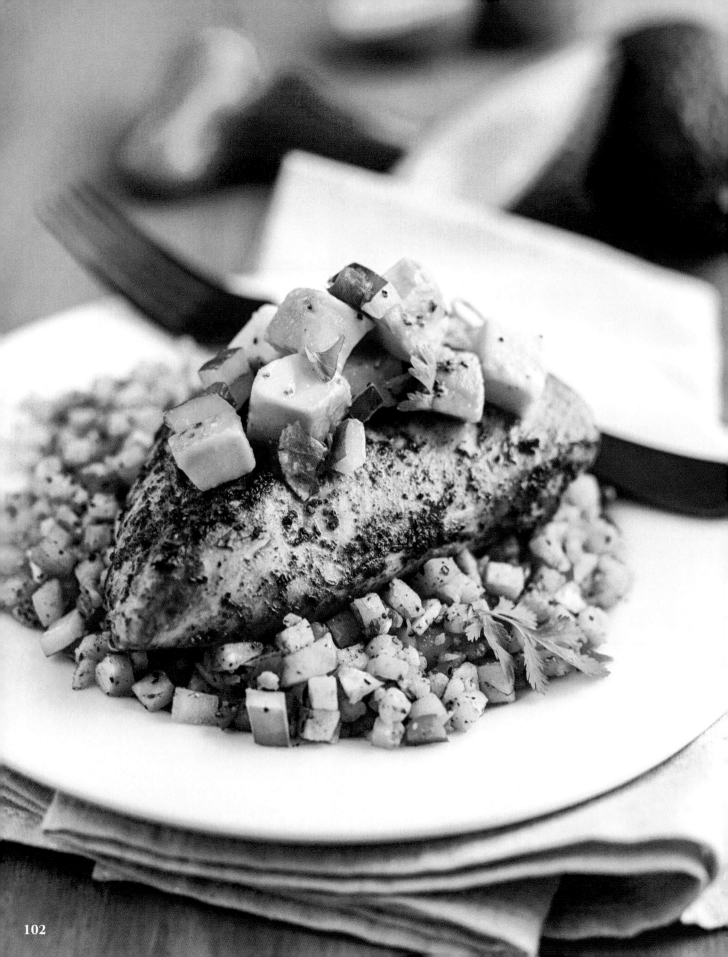

CHILI-RUBBED CHICKEN BREASTS
WITH CHOPPED GUACAMOLE

This chicken brings a bit of spice, but it isn't anything the cooling avocado in the Chopped Guacamole can't tame! The bold flavors and beautiful presentation may seem complicated, but this recipe is anything but.

SHOPPING LIST

4 boneless, skinless chicken breasts

1 tablespoon olive oil

1 tablespoon chili powder

1 teaspoon ground cumin

½ teaspoon salt

½ teaspoon black pepper

⅛ teaspoon ground cayenne pepper

CHOPPED GUACAMOLE

1 Hass avocado, pitted, peeled, and chopped

3 tablespoons diced red onion

3 tablespoons chopped cilantro

Juice of 1 lime

Salt and black pepper

1 HEAT a large skillet over medium-high heat.

2 IN a mixing bowl, toss chicken breasts with olive oil, chili powder, cumin, salt, pepper, and cayenne, until well coated.

3 PLACE seasoned chicken breasts in the hot skillet, and brown well, about 5 minutes on each side. Slice into the thickest chicken breast to ensure it is cooked throughout.

4 MEANWHILE, add all Chopped Guacamole ingredients to a mixing bowl, and toss to mix. Season to taste with salt and pepper.

5 TOP each chicken breast with an equal amount of the Chopped Guacamole to serve.

HELPFUL TIPS

Reducing the chili powder to 2 teaspoons, and omitting the ground cayenne pepper will make this milder spice-wise.

POULTRY

WHAT MAKES IT QUICK & EASY: By preparing the Chopped Guacamole as the chicken is cooking, you can save at least 5 minutes of prep time.

Calories: 300 • Fat: 15g • Protein: 40g • Total Carbs: 5g – Fiber: 3.5g = **Net Carbs: 1.5g**

CHICKEN SAUSAGE ITALIANO
WITH FRESH TOMATO SAUCE

My local grocery store now stocks a wonderful assortment of chicken sausages that are actually fresh and raw, not cured like hot dogs. This simple recipe can put them to great use in a fresh and delicate tomato sauce that is only lightly cooked.

SHOPPING LIST

1 tablespoon olive oil

5 fresh (raw) links Italian chicken sausage (see tip)

¼ cup diced yellow onion

2 teaspoons minced garlic

¼ cup water

2 tomatoes, diced

2 tablespoons chopped fresh basil

2 teaspoons balsamic vinegar

¼ teaspoon onion powder

¼ teaspoon garlic powder

Salt and black pepper

HELPFUL TIPS

Many grocery stores sell fresh chicken sausage now, however pre-cooked chicken sausage (sold near the hot dogs) can be used in a pinch.

1 HEAT olive oil in a large skillet over medium-high heat.

2 PLACE chicken sausage in the hot skillet and brown on all sides.

3 ADD onions to the skillet and sauté 1 minute, just until onions sweat.

4 ADD the water to the skillet, cover, and reduce heat to medium-low. Let simmer for 7 minutes.

5 ADD all remaining ingredients to the skillet and stir to combine.

6 BRING up to a simmer and let cook for 5 minutes. Season with salt and pepper to taste before serving.

WHAT MAKES IT QUICK & EASY: A fresh, lightly cooked tomato sauce like this one not only tastes vibrant, but saves you the (sometimes) hours of simmering traditional sauce.

Calories: 230 • Fat: 12g • Protein: 21.5g • Total Carbs: 4g – Fiber: 1g = **Net Carbs: 3g**

POULTRY

ROASTED PEPPER TURKEY MEATLOAF
WITH A TANGY TOMATO TOPPING

There are two main complaints with ground turkey: that it lacks moistness, and that it lacks flavor. I've solved both complaints in this meatloaf recipe by mixing roasted red peppers right into the meat. These pickled peppers pack both the flavor and moisture a meatloaf needs.

SHOPPING LIST

Nonstick cooking spray

MEATLOAF

2 pounds ground turkey

2 large eggs, beaten

2/3 cup grated Parmesan cheese

1/3 cup diced roasted red peppers (see tip)

1 tablespoon minced garlic

1½ teaspoons dried oregano

¾ teaspoon salt

¾ teaspoon black pepper

TOPPING

2 tablespoons tomato paste

1 tablespoon Dijon mustard

1 tablespoon water

1 PREHEAT oven to 375°F. Spray a 9x5-inch loaf pan with nonstick cooking spray.

2 IN a large mixing bowl, use your hands to combine all Meatloaf ingredients.

3 TRANSFER the meatloaf mixture to the prepared baking dish, and use your hands to form an even top.

4 WHISK together all Topping ingredients, and spread a thin layer over the top of the loaf.

5 BAKE for 55–60 minutes, or until a meat thermometer inserted into the loaf registers 165°F. Let rest 5 minutes before slicing.

HELPFUL TIPS

You can find diced or chopped roasted red peppers near the pickles in the grocery store. Diced pimentos will also work.

POULTRY

WHAT MAKES IT QUICK & EASY: This loaf can be prepared in advance, covered, and refrigerated until ready to bake.

Calories: 380 • Fat: 22g • Protein: 49.5g • Total Carbs: 2.5g – Fiber: 0g = **Net Carbs: 2.5g**

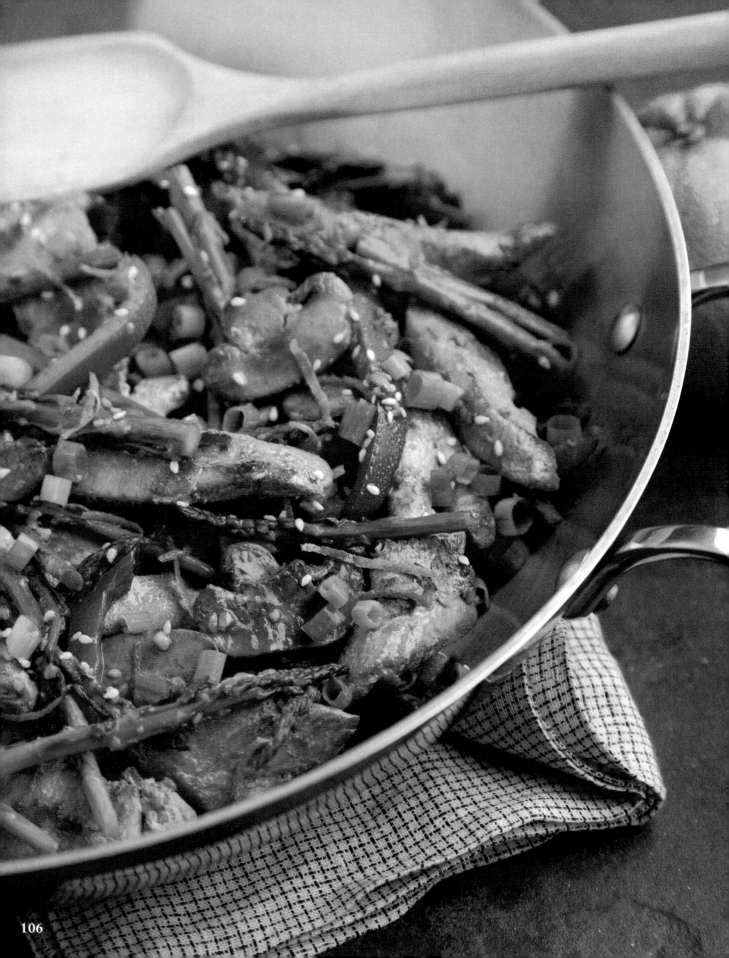

ORANGE CHICKEN STIR-FRY
WITH ASPARAGUS AND FIVE SPICE POWDER

Chinese five spice powder is a true essential in my spice armory. Much like curry, the combination of spices (star anise, clove, cinnamon, Sichuan pepper, and fennel) is far greater than their individual flavors. Many of these spices are often used in desserts as well, which is probably why they pair so well with orange zest in this savory stir-fry.

SHOPPING LIST

1 tablespoon vegetable oil

1¼ pounds boneless, skinless chicken breast, sliced

1 small bunch asparagus, cut into 3-inch lengths

8 ounces sliced mushrooms

½ red bell pepper, thinly sliced

3 tablespoons soy sauce

1 tablespoon orange zest

2 teaspoons minced garlic

1 teaspoon sugar substitute

1 teaspoon five spice powder (see tip)

6 green onions, thinly sliced

1 HEAT oil in a large skillet or wok over high heat until nearly smoking hot.

2 ADD the sliced chicken to the hot skillet. Sauté until golden brown, about 5 minutes.

3 REDUCE heat to medium-high. Add all remaining ingredients, except green onions, to the skillet and sauté for 7 minutes, stirring constantly, until asparagus is crisp-tender.

4 STIR in sliced green onions before serving.

POULTRY

HELPFUL TIPS

Five spice powder can be found in either the spice aisle or Asian foods section of the grocery store.

WHAT MAKES IT QUICK & EASY: Stir-fry always makes for a quick one-pot meal.

Calories: 220 · Fat: 5g · Protein: 37.5g · Total Carbs: 9.5g – Fiber: 3.5g = **Net Carbs: 6g**

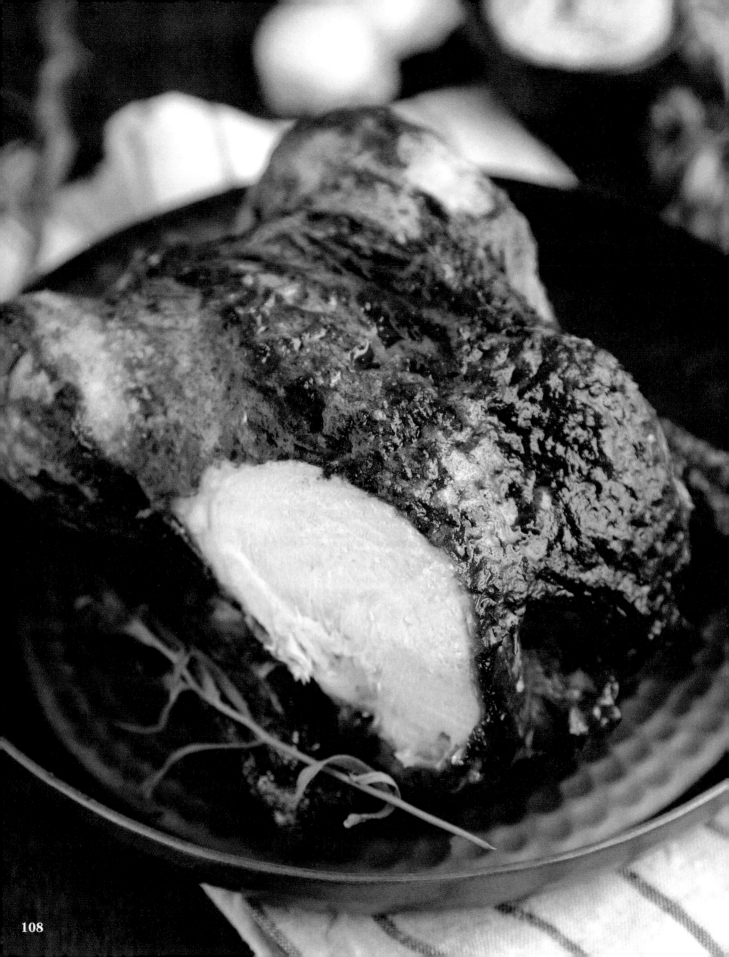

WHOLE ROASTED CHICKEN

WITH DIJON AND TARRAGON

There are few things simpler than a whole roasted chicken… However, preparing one can be daunting for some. I'm here to say that it is not only easy, but it is an everyday recipe that every cook should have in their rotation. Nutritional information is for ¼ of all meat (both white and dark) and skin of the cooked chicken.

SHOPPING LIST

1 (4-pound) roasting chicken, giblets removed

4 cloves garlic, peeled and halved

2 sprigs tarragon

2 tablespoons unsalted butter, melted

2 tablespoons Dijon mustard

1 tablespoon chopped fresh tarragon

2 teaspoons minced garlic

¼ teaspoon salt

HELPFUL TIPS

Tarragon has a licorice-type flavor that some may not like. In this instance, sprigs and chopped fresh thyme can be used for a more classic flavor.

POULTRY

1 PREHEAT oven to 400°F.

2 PLACE chicken in a roasting pan, and stuff garlic and sprigs of tarragon into the cavity.

3 IN a small bowl, use a fork to whisk together butter, Dijon mustard, tarragon, minced garlic, and salt. Spread over the entire surface of the chicken.

4 BAKE for 1 hour 15 minutes before checking with a meat thermometer inserted near the bone of the thigh. The chicken is done when the temperature registers 175°F.

5 LET rest at least 10 minutes before carving.

WHAT MAKES IT QUICK & EASY: Most recipes for whole chickens take 30 minutes longer at 350°F, but 400°F is the sweet spot for speed, moist meat, and crispy skin.

Calories: 600 • Fat: 37g • Protein: 62.5g • Total Carbs: 1g – Fiber: 0g = **Net Carbs: 1g**

CURRY CHICKEN THIGHS

SWEET, SPICY, AND FLAVORFUL ROASTED CHICKEN

Indian food takeout can take a night off with this recipe for boldly seasoned boneless, skinless chicken thighs. Unlike many Indian dishes, these are not stewed, but roasted to really toast all of those wonderful spices.

SHOPPING LIST

Nonstick cooking spray

8 boneless, skinless chicken thighs (about 2 pounds)

1 tablespoon vegetable oil

2 teaspoons curry powder

1 teaspoon sugar substitute, optional

½ teaspoon salt

¼ teaspoon ground cumin

¼ teaspoon ground cayenne pepper

1 PREHEAT oven to 400°F. Spray a sheet pan with nonstick cooking spray.

2 IN a mixing bowl, toss chicken thighs with all remaining ingredients, coating well. Transfer to the prepared sheet pan.

3 BAKE for 25–30 minutes, or until cutting into the largest thigh reveals juices that run clear.

HELPFUL TIPS

This can also be made with chicken breasts in place of the thighs by lowering the oven temperature to 375°F.

WHAT MAKES IT QUICK & EASY: With a well-stocked spice rack, this recipe can be made with a shopping list of only 1 ingredient (the chicken thighs).

Calories: 305 • Fat: 12g • Protein: 44g • Total Carbs: 1g − Fiber: 0g = **Net Carbs: 1g**

POULTRY

CHICKEN CORDON BLEU SKILLET
WITH BROCCOLI

All the flavors of Chicken Cordon Bleu are sautéed together in this quick entrée skillet. Whole grain mustard adds a nice bite to the chicken, ham, and broccoli, without adding as much spice as a mustard like Dijon. For the final touch, melted Swiss cheese tops it all off.

SHOPPING LIST

2 tablespoons unsalted butter

3 boneless, skinless chicken breasts, cut into 1-inch cubes

Salt and black pepper

8 ounces cubed ham

1 (12-ounce) bag frozen broccoli florets

¼ cup chicken stock

1 tablespoon whole grain mustard

¼ teaspoon onion powder

4 slices Swiss cheese

HELPFUL TIPS

I like to make this with cubed boneless, skinless chicken thighs as well, as they are just about guaranteed to be tender.

1 HEAT butter in a large skillet over medium-high heat, until sizzling.

2 GENEROUSLY season cubed chicken with salt and pepper.

3 PLACE seasoned chicken in the hot skillet, and cook, stirring occasionally, until browned on all sides, about 5 minutes.

4 STIR all remaining ingredients, except Swiss cheese, into the skillet, and bring up to a simmer.

5 REDUCE heat to medium-low, cover, and let cook for 5 minutes, or until broccoli is heated through.

6 TOP all with the 4 slices of Swiss cheese; cover, and cook for 1 additional minute to melt cheese. Serve immediately.

POULTRY

WHAT MAKES IT QUICK & EASY: Using frozen broccoli florets allows you to make this in one skillet without overcooking the chicken.

Calories: 370 • Fat: 16.5g • Protein: 49g • Total Carbs: 8g – Fiber: 2g = **Net Carbs: 6g**

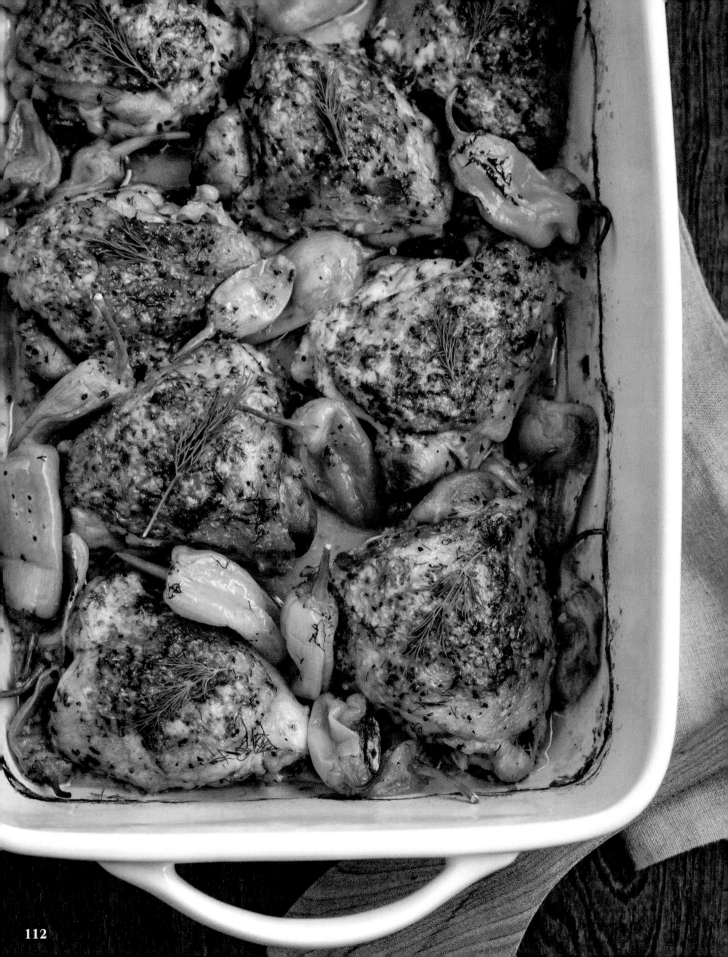

MISSISSIPPI ROAST CHICKEN THIGHS

MY TAKE ON AN INTERNET PHENOMENON

Mississippi Roast or simply "Roast" was created by a woman named Robin Chapman many years ago, but has recently gone on to become one of the most popular recipes online. Variations on the beef roast with pepperoncini peppers and ranch flavoring can be found all over, so I set out to develop something a little different. I've used chicken thighs and fresh ingredients rather than beef and powdered seasonings to retain the spirit of Chapman's creation, while also making it my own.

SHOPPING LIST

1 tablespoon vegetable oil

8 chicken thighs (about 3 pounds)

Salt and black pepper

1 (16-ounce) jar pepperoncinis, drained well

2 tablespoons chopped fresh dill

½ cup ranch dressing (see tip)

HELPFUL TIPS

We recommend using a refrigerated brand of ranch dressing (sold in the produce section), as they do not have MSG. Look for a brand with 1g of carbs or less.

1 PREHEAT oven to 325°F.

2 HEAT vegetable oil in a large skillet over medium-high heat.

3 GENEROUSLY season chicken thighs with salt and pepper.

4 PLACE chicken into the skillet and cook on both sides until skin is well browned. Transfer to a large baking dish, skin-side up.

5 ADD the pepperoncinis to the baking dish, surrounding the chicken. Sprinkle dill over top of all.

6 TOP each chicken thigh with 2 tablespoons of the ranch dressing.

7 COVER and bake for 1 hour.

8 UNCOVER and bake an additional 30 minutes, or until ranch dressing has melted into the chicken skin and browned. Serve chicken thighs with the pepperoncinis. Lightly drizzle with juices from the baking dish to keep the meat moist.

POULTRY

WHAT MAKES IT QUICK & EASY: While the cook time is long to make for the most tender meat, the prep is done in only minutes and with only a handful of ingredients.

Calories: 525 · Fat: 40g · Protein: 32.5g · Total Carbs: 3.5g − Fiber: 0g = **Net Carbs: 3.5g**

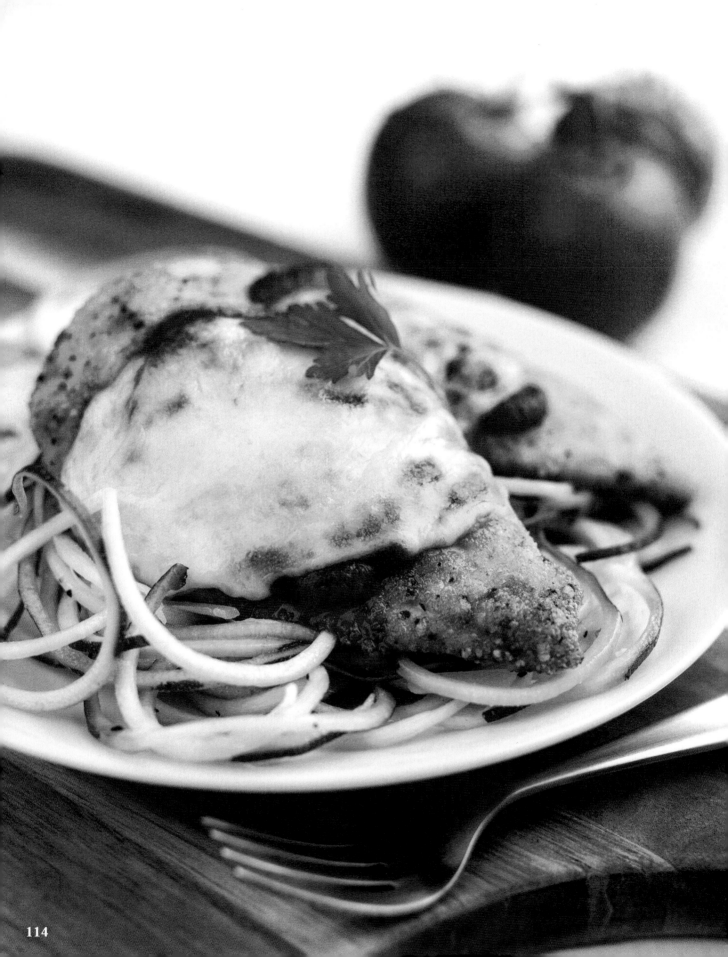

CHICKEN PARMESAN

A LOW-CARB RENAISSANCE FOR AN ITALIAN CLASSIC

Chicken Parmesan is about as classic a comfort food as you get. I've reinvented it in the past without the breading—but let's face it—we all want that breading! Finally, I've created a low-carb breading that browns well, tastes great, and is far more simple than you'd ever think… In fact, that breading you see in the picture is only Parmesan cheese and spices. Sometimes, the simplest solutions are also the best. Serve over one of my Pasta Alternatives, recipes page: 170.

SHOPPING LIST

2 large eggs

¼ teaspoon salt

¼ teaspoon garlic powder

1 cup grated Parmesan cheese

1 teaspoon Italian seasoning

4 boneless, skinless chicken breasts

¼ teaspoon black pepper

2 tablespoons olive oil

⅓ cup prepared pasta sauce

¾ cup shredded mozzarella cheese or 4 slices provolone cheese

HELPFUL TIPS

Thinner chicken breasts work best in this recipe. I've noticed that boneless chicken breasts are now sometimes as large as 12 ounces each! What are they feeding those chickens? For a monster cut like that, you should lay plastic wrap over the breasts and pound with a mallet or rolling pin until 1-inch thick.

POULTRY

1 PREHEAT oven to 375°F.

2 IN a shallow but wide bowl, whisk eggs with salt and garlic powder to create an egg wash.

3 IN a separate bowl, combine Parmesan cheese with Italian seasoning to create a breading.

4 DIP chicken breasts in the egg wash, flipping to thoroughly coat. Transfer to the breading mixture, and press the chicken into the cheese to ensure the breading adheres.

5 HEAT olive oil in a large skillet over medium-high heat.

6 PLACE the breaded chicken breasts in the skillet, and cook for 4–5 minutes on each side, just until the breading is golden brown.

7 TRANSFER the browned chicken breasts to a sheet pan, and top each with an equal amount of the pasta sauce, then an equal amount of mozzarella cheese.

8 BAKE for 10 minutes, just until cheese has melted, and slicing into the largest chicken breast reveals no pink.

WHAT MAKES IT QUICK & EASY: This is a made-from-scratch comfort food dinner you can have on your table in only a little over 30 minutes.

Calories: 375 · Fat: 18g · Protein: 55g · Total Carbs: 2.5g – Fiber: 0g = **Net Carbs: 2.5g**

GIANT BUFFALO DRUMSTICKS

FULL-SIZED DRUMSTICKS, BUFFALO-STYLE

There's only one problem with Buffalo wings—even though they are named as if they're large—they're just never big enough…at least, if you love wings as much as I do! I've solved this dilemma of mine by making Giant Buffalo Drumsticks from full-sized chicken legs.

SHOPPING LIST

Nonstick cooking spray

8 chicken legs (not drumettes)

Salt and black pepper

Garlic powder

3 tablespoons unsalted butter, melted

2 tablespoons Louisiana hot sauce

HELPFUL TIPS

Like any Buffalo wing, you've gotta serve these alongside my Blue Cheese Dressing, recipe page: 50.

1 PREHEAT oven to 450°F. Line a sheet pan with aluminum foil and spray foil with nonstick cooking spray.

2 PLACE chicken legs on the prepared sheet pan and season.

3 IN a large mixing bowl, toss chicken legs with all remaining ingredients.

4 TRANSFER the coated legs to the prepared sheet pan, and season generously with salt, pepper, and garlic powder.

5 BAKE for 35 minutes, flipping halfway through. Chicken legs are done when a meat thermometer inserted into the thickest part registers 175°F.

6 IN a large mixing bowl, whisk together butter and hot sauce. Add the cooked chicken legs to the bowl, and toss to coat in the sauce. Serve immediately.

WHAT MAKES IT QUICK & EASY: While these are pretty easy to make, they're far easier to eat (with far more meat) than tiny drumettes.

Calories: 605 · Fat: 39.5g · Protein: 59g · Total Carbs: 0g – Fiber: 0g = **Net Carbs: 0g**

POULTRY

GRILLED ITALIAN CHICKEN

MARINATED CHICKEN, GRILLED UP MOIST

With this recipe, there's no need to go hunting for Italian dressings or marinades that don't contain a laundry list of foreign ingredients (they're very hard to find). Whisking up your own Italian marinade is not only easy, but much more flavorful than anything that has a several-year shelf-life.

SHOPPING LIST

4 boneless, skinless chicken breasts

MARINADE

⅓ cup extra-virgin olive oil

⅓ cup red wine vinegar

2 tablespoons minced red onion

1 tablespoon minced garlic

1 tablespoon Italian seasoning

¾ teaspoon salt

¾ teaspoon black pepper

HELPFUL TIPS

While these are best when marinated for at least 2 hours, you should not leave the chicken in the marinade for more than 12 hours, as the acid in the vinegar will eventually break down the meat. Yes, there is such a thing as TOO tender!

1 PLACE chicken breasts in a bowl or food storage container, and top with all marinade ingredients, tossing to mix.

2 COVER and refrigerate for at least 2 hours, to marinate.

3 OIL a grill or grill pan and preheat on high heat.

4 REMOVE chicken breasts from marinade, discarding used marinade.

5 GRILL chicken breasts for 6–8 minutes on each side, or until slicing into the thickest part reveals no pink.

POULTRY

WHAT MAKES IT QUICK & EASY: With a well-stocked pantry, this recipe can be made with a shopping list of only 1 ingredient (the chicken breasts.

Calories: 240 · Fat: 9.5g · Protein: 39g · Total Carbs: 1g – Fiber: 0g = **Net Carbs: 1g**

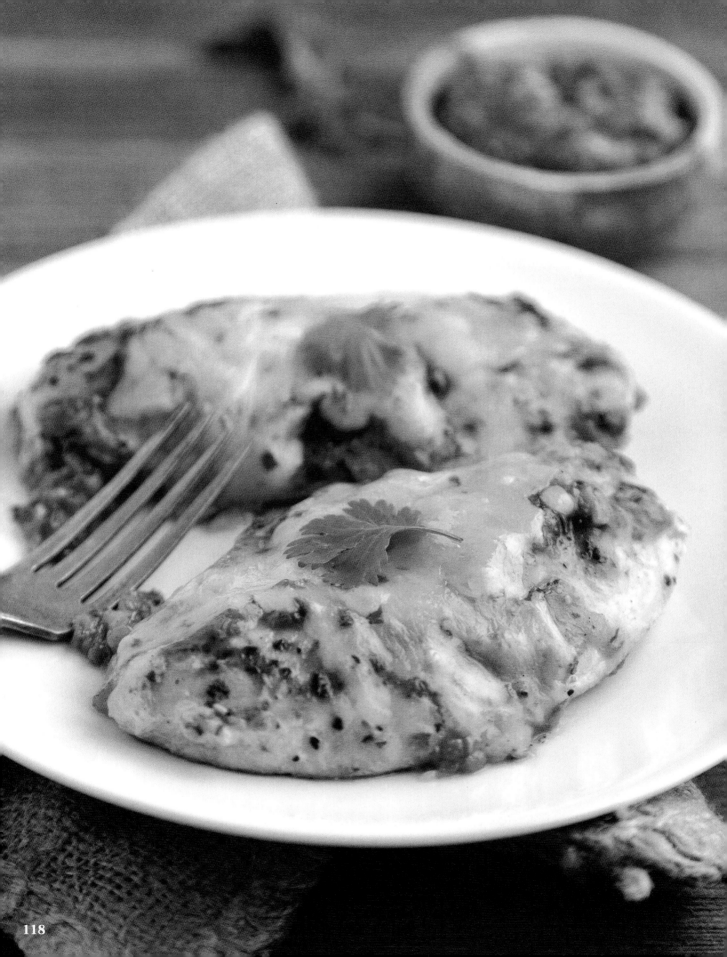

RECAITO CHICKEN

CHICKEN WITH CULANTRO SAUCE AND PEPPER-JACK CHEESE

Recaito is a Puerto Rican cooking base that looks very similar to salsa verde. Made from blended bell pepper, onion, garlic, and culantro (which is closely related to cilantro), recaito is often used as a flavorful starter for stews. Here, I've used it to give these chicken breasts a ton of flavor, using very few ingredients.

SHOPPING LIST

2 teaspoons olive oil

4 boneless, skinless chicken breasts

Salt and black pepper

Garlic powder

½ cup recaito (see tip)

⅔ cup shredded pepper-jack cheese

HELPFUL TIPS

You can find jars of recaito in either the ethnic foods section near the salsas, or in the spice aisle near products by the brand Goya.

1 HEAT oil in a large skillet over medium-high heat.

2 GENEROUSLY season chicken breasts with salt, pepper, and garlic powder.

3 PLACE seasoned chicken breasts in the hot skillet and brown well, about 5 minutes on each side. Slice into the thickest chicken breast to ensure it is cooked throughout.

4 REDUCE heat to low and add recaito to the skillet. Toss chicken breasts in the recaito to fully coat.

5 TOP each chicken breast with an equal amount of the pepper-jack cheese. Cover skillet and let cook for 1 minute to melt the cheese. Serve immediately.

POULTRY

WHAT MAKES IT QUICK & EASY: For a recipe with so much flavor, it's hard to believe it can be made with so few ingredients, in so little time.

Calories: 260 • Fat: 10g • Protein: 44g • Total Carbs: 1.5g − Fiber: 0g = **Net Carbs: 1.5g**

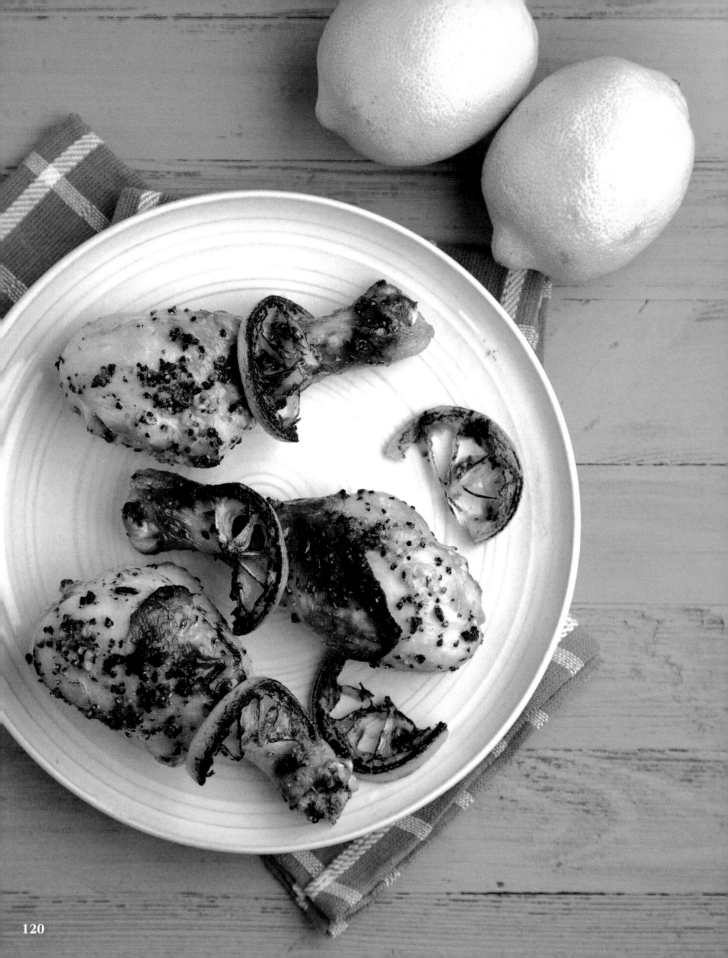

LEMON & GARLIC CHICKEN LEGS

ZESTY CHICKEN DRUMSTICKS

Lemon and garlic are a timeless duo that pairs perfectly with chicken. Here, I've paired this dynamic duo with roasted chicken legs for moist dark meat that literally falls off the bone.

SHOPPING LIST

Nonstick cooking spray

8 chicken legs (not drumettes)

1 tablespoon olive oil

Zest of 1 lemon

Juice of ½ lemon

1 tablespoon minced garlic

½ teaspoon salt

½ teaspoon black pepper

HELPFUL TIPS

For a nice presentation you can roast lemon slices, as pictured, by placing thick-sliced lemon on the sheet pan when flipping the chicken legs halfway through cooking.

1 PREHEAT oven to 450°F. Line a sheet pan with aluminum foil and spray foil with nonstick cooking spray.

2 IN a large mixing bowl, toss chicken legs with all remaining ingredients.

3 TRANSFER the coated legs to the prepared sheet pan.

4 BAKE for 35 minutes, flipping halfway through. Chicken legs are done when a meat thermometer inserted into the thickest part registers 175°F.

POULTRY

WHAT MAKES IT QUICK & EASY: This recipe gives you all the flavor of chicken that has been marinated, without all the wait.

Calories: 540 • Fat: 32g • Protein: 59g • Total Carbs: 1g − Fiber: 0g = **Net Carbs: 1g**

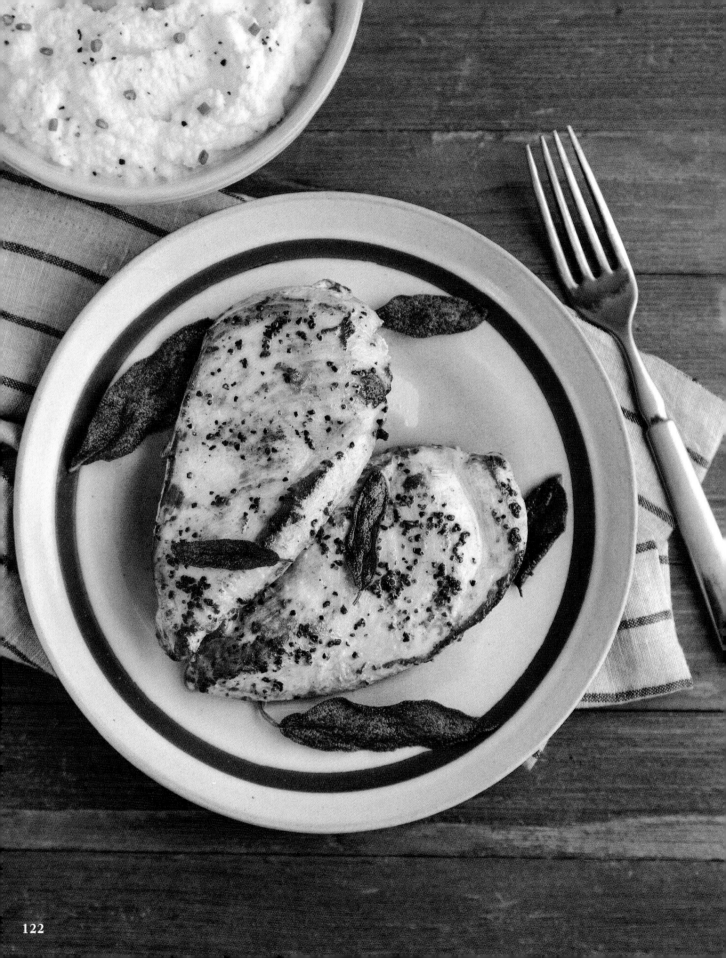

BROWN BUTTER CHICKEN
WITH CRISPY SAGE

Something amazing happens to butter as it browns… It takes on a very complex and nutty flavor that is one of the simplest, but best tasting sauces you can make. Adding sage to the butter makes for a classic sauce that has and will continue to stand the test of time— and taste!

SHOPPING LIST

2 teaspoons vegetable oil

4 boneless, skinless chicken breasts

Salt and black pepper

4 tablespoons unsalted butter

8 leaves sage

HELPFUL TIPS

It's best to brown the butter in a pan that is silver (not nonstick), as you can better see the color of the butter as it browns. The perfect color is seen in the photo at left.

1 HEAT oil in a large skillet over medium-high heat, until nearly smoking hot.

2 GENEROUSLY season the chicken breasts with salt and pepper before adding to the hot skillet.

3 COOK chicken until well browned and slicing into the thickest piece reveals no pink, about 5 minutes on each side.

4 MEANWHILE, place butter and sage in a second, smaller skillet over medium heat.

5 LET butter and sage cook, stirring occasionally, for the full 10 minutes the chicken is cooking, or until butter is a rich golden brown color.

6 SERVE chicken topped with crispy sage and drizzled with brown butter.

POULTRY

WHAT MAKES IT QUICK & EASY: This is a restaurant-quality dish made with only a handful of ingredients.

Calories: 285 • Fat: 15g • Protein: 39g • Total Carbs: 0.5g – Fiber: 0g = **Net Carbs: 0.5g**

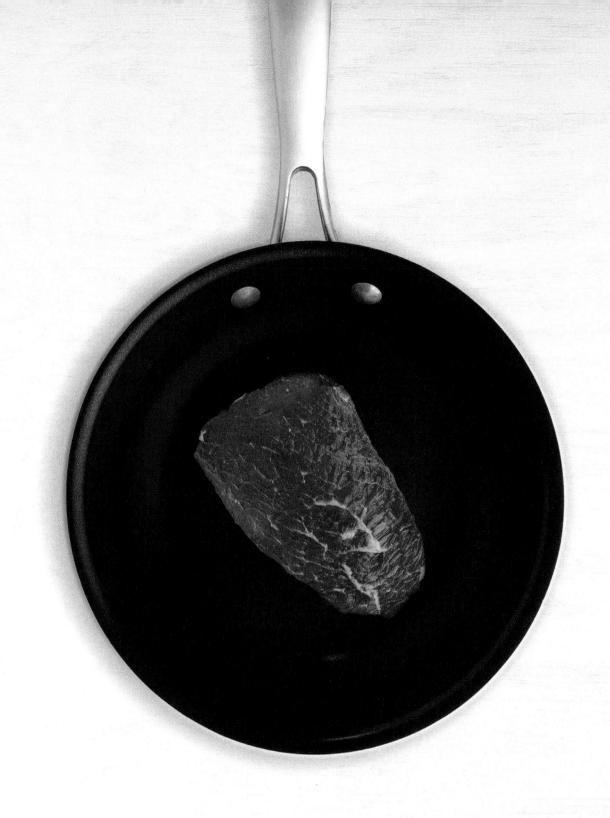

MEATS

MEATS

QUICK & EASY COMPOUND BUTTERS

DIRECTIONS

EACH RECIPE MAKES ABOUT 10 (1-TABLESPOON) SERVINGS

1 IN a blender or food processor, combine all ingredients, lightly blending, just until combined.

2 SPOON the butter onto a piece of plastic wrap and form into a thick log. Roll the plastic wrap into a cylinder and twist the ends shut. For an even nicer presentation, you can spoon the butter into silicone molds. Many molds work well, including mini loaf molds, food-grade soap molds, or even silicone muffin pans. Spread the butter into the molds and tap against the counter to remove any air bubbles.

3 REFRIGERATE for at least 1 hour before unwrapping or unmolding. Compound butters freeze well for longterm storage.

"THESE FLAVORED BUTTERS ARE PERFECT FOR SERVING OVER MEATS OR VEGETABLES. YOU CAN ALSO USE THEM IN PLACE OF REGULAR BUTTER WHEN COOKING TO SPRUCE UP ANY DISH."

CILANTRO-LIME BUTTER

GREAT OVER SEAFOOD, CHICKEN, OR PORK

½ cup (1 stick) unsalted butter, softened

3 tablespoons chopped cilantro

2 tablespoons minced shallots

Juice of 1 small lime

¾ teaspoon salt

¾ teaspoon black pepper

Calories: 85 • Fat: 9g • Protein: 0g
Total Carbs: 0.5g – Fiber: 0g = **Net Carbs: 0.5g**

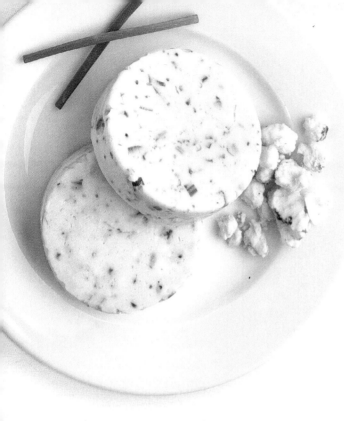

GORGONZOLA & CHIVE BUTTER

GREAT OVER STEAK OR CHICKEN

½ cup (1 stick) unsalted butter, softened

¼ cup crumbled Gorgonzola cheese

2 tablespoons chopped chives

½ teaspoon Worcestershire sauce

½ teaspoon salt

½ teaspoon black pepper

Calories: 95 • Fat: 10.5g • Protein: 1g
Total Carbs: 0.5g – Fiber: 0g = **Net Carbs: 0.5g**

KALAMATA OLIVE BUTTER

GREAT OVER SEAFOOD OR CHICKEN

½ cup (1 stick) unsalted butter, softened

¼ cup Kalamata olives

1 tablespoon chopped fresh oregano

2 teaspoons minced garlic

1 teaspoon lemon juice

1 teaspoon lemon zest

¼ teaspoon black pepper

Calories: 90 • Fat: 9.5g • Protein: 0g
Total Carbs: 1g – Fiber: 0g = **Net Carbs: 1g**

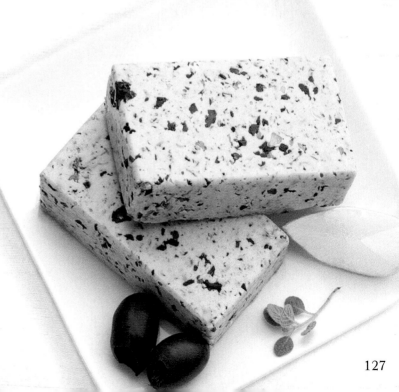

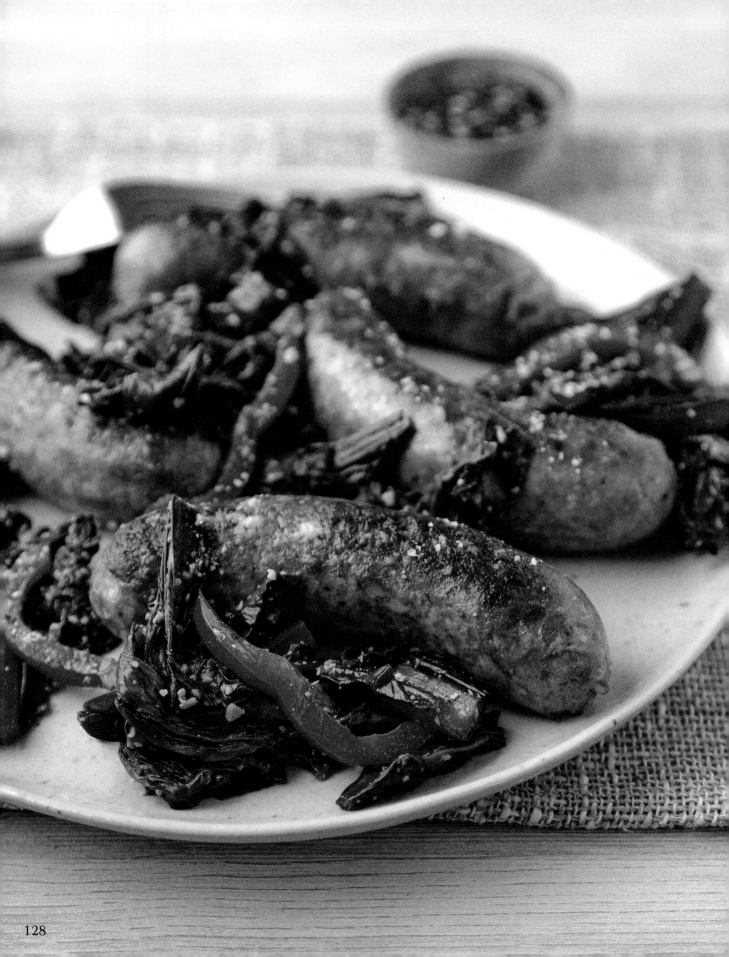

ITALIAN SAUSAGE WITH SWISS CHARD

SAUSAGE WITH SWEET GREENS AND BELL PEPPER

Flavorful one-skillet meals made in thirty minutes or less always seem to be in high demand. These Italian sausages meet those standards on their own, complemented by the sweet earthiness of Swiss chard and sliced bell pepper, but if you're really hungry, they can be served alongside Spaghetti Squash, recipe page: 170.

SHOPPING LIST

1 tablespoon olive oil

5 fresh (raw) links Italian sausage

¼ cup water

1 bunch Swiss chard, ends trimmed, chopped large

½ red bell pepper, thinly sliced

2 teaspoons white wine vinegar

2 teaspoons minced garlic

1 teaspoon sugar substitute, optional

¼ teaspoon salt

¼ teaspoon black pepper

2 tablespoons grated Parmesan cheese

HELPFUL TIPS

For a bit of spice, hot Italian sausage can be used and a pinch of crushed red pepper flakes can be added to the Swiss chard while sautéing.

1 HEAT olive oil in a large skillet over medium-high heat.

2 PLACE Italian sausage in the hot skillet and brown on all sides.

3 ADD water to the skillet, cover, and reduce heat to medium-low. Let simmer for 7 minutes.

4 REMOVE sausages from skillet, cover, and set aside.

5 PLACE Swiss chard, bell pepper, vinegar, garlic, sugar substitute, salt, and pepper in the skillet and sauté until chard has cooked down, about 5 minutes.

6 RETURN the sausages to the skillet and toss with the chard, cooking just 1 minute to reheat.

7 REMOVE from heat and sprinkle with Parmesan cheese before serving.

MEATS

WHAT MAKES IT QUICK & EASY: Typically, you'd boil the sausage before browning, however this recipe does everything in one skillet.

Calories: 280 • Fat: 21.5g • Protein: 19g • Total Carbs: 3g − Fiber: 1g = **Net Carbs: 2g**

PAN-SEARED LONDON BROIL

WITH OR WITHOUT COMPOUND BUTTER

This basic recipe for London Broil offers the chance to try any of my Compound Butters, recipe page: 126. Searing the steak in a cast-iron skillet makes for a beautifully-browned crust without having to light up the grill… Or clean it after cooking!

SHOPPING LIST

1 tablespoon vegetable oil

1 tablespoon unsalted butter

1 (2½-pound) London broil steak (1 inch thick)

Salt and black pepper

Garlic Powder

2 tablespoons Compound Butter, recipe page: 126, if desired

HELPFUL TIPS

When cooking steaks, it is better to let them sit out for about 10 minutes before cooking. Most chefs let them come to room temperature (sitting out over 30 minutes), as they cook more evenly that way. I don't explicitly recommend that, but letting them sit out as you prep is better than nothing (and safer than 30 minutes or more).

1 HEAT vegetable oil and butter in a cast-iron skillet over medium-high heat.

2 GENEROUSLY season both sides of the steak with salt, pepper, and garlic powder.

3 BROWN the steak well, about 4 minutes on each side for medium-rare.

4 REMOVE skillet from heat and top steak with your choice of Compound Butter, if desired. Let steak rest in pan for 4 minutes as the heat of the pan continues to cook it without over-browning, and the compound butter melts.

5 USE a meat thermometer to check for doneness, ensuring it registers 140°F for medium-rare. If the steak is not up to temperature, return to the heat for 1–2 additional minutes.

6 TRANSFER steak to a cutting board, tent with aluminum foil, and let rest for 5 additional minutes before thinly slicing against the grain.

WHAT MAKES IT QUICK & EASY: By keeping Compound Butter in your freezer, you can always have a flavorful steak, without having to buy a full basket of ingredients.

Calories: 450 • Fat: 32g • Protein: 38.5g • Total Carbs: 0g − Fiber: 0g = **Net Carbs: 0g**

PORK WITH CHICKEN GRAVY

LOIN CHOPS WITH A CREAMY CRACKED PEPPER GRAVY

There is something so addictive about good gravy… Sometimes you may find yourself wanting to pour the whole boat onto your plate. The gravy over these pork chops is so good, you're gonna' need a bigger boat. I like to serve this over my Cauliflower Rice, recipe page: 173.

SHOPPING LIST

2 teaspoons vegetable oil

8 boneless pork loin chops (about 2 pounds)

Salt and black pepper

Garlic powder

CHICKEN GRAVY

½ cup heavy cream

1 teaspoon chicken base

½ teaspoon cracked black pepper

¼ teaspoon onion powder

2 tablespoons unsalted butter

Salt

HELPFUL TIPS

Chicken base can be purchased in small jars near the stocks and broths in the grocery store. Because it is concentrated, you can add far more chicken flavor than simply adding stock.

1 HEAT oil in a large skillet over medium-high heat, until nearly smoking hot.

2 GENEROUSLY season pork chops with salt, pepper, and garlic powder. Add the seasoned pork chops to the hot skillet and brown well, about 4 minutes on each side. Remove from pan and let rest 5 minutes.

3 MEANWHILE, in a small sauce pot over medium heat, whisk together heavy cream, chicken base, pepper, and onion powder. Bring up to a slow simmer.

4 REMOVE gravy from heat and stir in butter to slightly thicken. Season with salt to taste.

5 SERVE rested pork chops with the Chicken Gravy drizzled over top.

MEATS

WHAT MAKES IT QUICK & EASY: Using chicken base in this recipe allows you to develop flavors without having to reduce chicken stock for 15 or more minutes.

Calories: 445 • Fat: 21.5g • Protein: 60g • Total Carbs: 0.5g – Fiber: 0g = **Net Carbs: 0.5g**

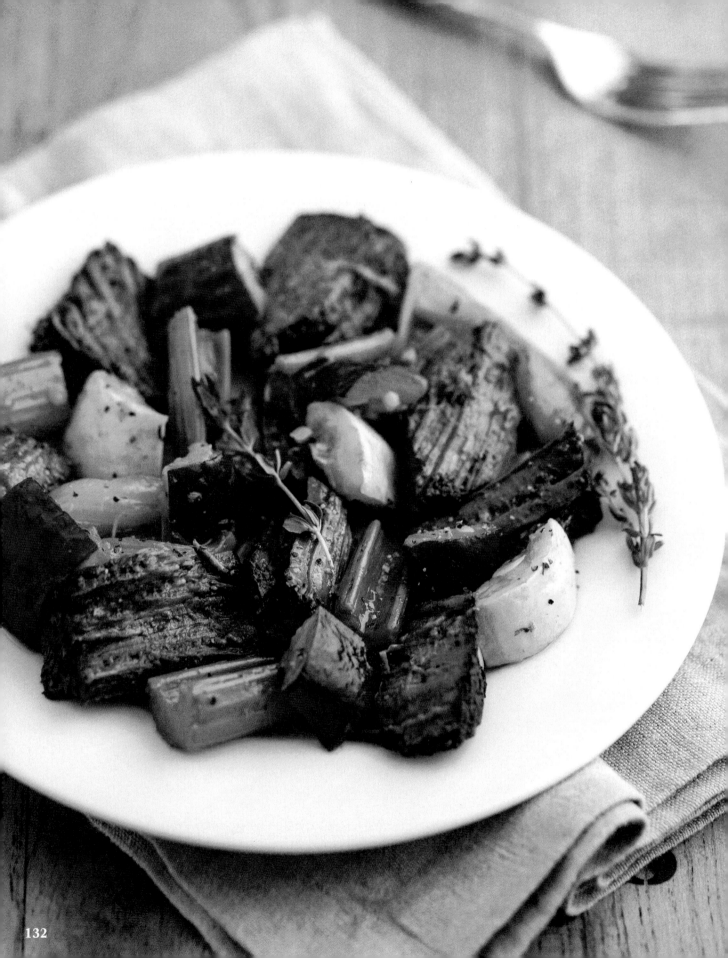

2-HOUR POT ROAST

WITH ZUCCHINI AND YELLOW SQUASH

I'm pushing the limits of pot roast-cookery in this blazing fast take on the quintessential beef dinner. Yes, traditional pot roast takes so long to cook that I think I can say that 2 hours is "blazing fast" and get away with it!

SHOPPING LIST

1 tablespoon vegetable oil

1 tablespoon unsalted butter

1 boneless beef chuck roast (about 2½ pounds)

Salt and black pepper

Garlic powder

1 yellow onion, quartered

3 stalks celery, cut into 1-inch lengths

4 sprigs fresh thyme

2 bay leaves

1 large yellow squash, chopped

1 large zucchini, chopped

HELPFUL TIPS

For a creamier gravy, transfer pan juices to a saucepan and simmer rapidly, until reduced by about ⅓. Remove from heat and stir in 6 tablespoons of butter.

1 PREHEAT oven to 350°F.

2 HEAT vegetable oil and butter in a Dutch oven over high heat, until sizzling.

3 CUT chuck roast into 4 equal-sized pieces. Generously season the roast pieces with salt, pepper, and garlic powder.

4 PLACE seasoned roast in the hot Dutch oven and brown each piece on all sides.

5 REMOVE from heat and top the meat with the onion, celery, thyme, and bay leaves.

6 COVER and bake for 90 minutes.

7 UNCOVER and add the chopped squash and zucchini to the Dutch oven. Cover and bake an additional 30 minutes, or until meat is tender.

8 PULL apart meat to serve alongside vegetables. Season the juices from the pan to drizzle over top all.

MEATS

WHAT MAKES IT QUICK & EASY: By cutting the roast into 4 pieces, you can dramatically cut down on cook time.

Calories: 410 • Fat: 16g • Protein: 58.5g • Total Carbs: 5.5g – Fiber: 1.5g = **Net Carbs: 4g**

SERVES: 4

GROUND BEEF STROGANOFF
A CREAMY FAMILY-FAVORITE SKILLET MEAL

This classic dish deriving from a Russian recipe traditionally calls for hunks of beef to be braised slowly. I've removed the braising step in favor of ground beef to cut down on the cooking time. Instead of the egg noodles everyone has come to be so attached to, this creamy concoction is just as delicious when served over the top of one of my Pasta Alternatives, recipe page: 170.

SHOPPING LIST

1 tablespoon vegetable oil

1¼ pounds ground beef

1 teaspoon Worcestershire sauce

8 ounces sliced baby bella mushrooms

⅔ cup diced celery

⅓ cup chopped yellow onion

2 teaspoons minced garlic

1 cup sour cream

2 tablespoons fresh chopped tarragon

¾ teaspoon salt

½ teaspoon black pepper

½ teaspoon onion powder

HELPFUL TIPS

This can also be made with ground turkey or even ground pork.

1 HEAT oil in a large skillet over medium-high heat, until sizzling.

2 PLACE ground beef and Worcestershire sauce in the hot skillet and brown well, crumbling as it cooks.

3 DRAIN any excess grease from the skillet before adding mushrooms, celery, onion, and garlic.

4 SAUTÉ for 7 minutes, or until mushrooms are tender.

5 REMOVE from heat and stir in all remaining ingredients. Return to the heat, stirring constantly, just long enough for the sour cream to come to a simmer.

6 REMOVE from heat and let rest 3 minutes before serving.

WHAT MAKES IT QUICK & EASY: Traditional stroganoff is made with chunks of beef that must be braised for at least 30 minutes to become tender.

Calories: 540 · Fat: 37g · Protein: 43g · Total Carbs: 8g − Fiber: 1.5g = **Net Carbs: 6.5g**

BACON-WRAPPED BONELESS BBQ RIBS
COUNTRY-STYLE PORK RIBS WRAPPED IN MORE PORK

Country-style ribs are actually boneless cuts of lean pork and that can sometimes make for less than tender results, but wrapping them in bacon solves this issue by adding enough fat to make for wonderfully succulent meat…plus, you get to eat the actual bacon, which is always a good thing.

SHOPPING LIST

Nonstick cooking spray

8 boneless country-style pork ribs (about 2 pounds)

8 slices raw bacon

QUICK BBQ SAUCE

½ cup no-sugar-added ketchup

2 teaspoons smoked paprika

1 teaspoon Worcestershire sauce

½ teaspoon onion powder

½ teaspoon garlic powder

½ teaspoon black pepper

1 PREHEAT oven to 350°F. Line a sheet pan with aluminum foil sprayed with nonstick cooking spray.

2 PLACE ribs in a large mixing bowl. Add all Quick BBQ Sauce ingredients, and toss to mix and fully coat the meat. Transfer the coated ribs to the prepared sheet pan.

3 WRAP each rib with a slice of bacon, securing with toothpicks for best results.

4 BAKE for 40 minutes, or until bacon is crisp and pork mostly white throughout.

HELPFUL TIPS

As this cut of pork is very lean, these ribs will have the consistency of pork chops, however, you can cook them to be fall apart tender with a little more time. Simply bake uncovered for 20 minutes at 350°F, then cover, reduce temperature to 250°F for 1½ hours of cooking, or until desired tenderness.

MEATS

WHAT MAKES IT QUICK & EASY: This has all the flavor of ribs, only it is far easier to eat without the bones!

Calories: 455 • Fat: 23.5g • Protein: 50g • Total Carbs: 3g – Fiber: 0g = **Net Carbs: 3g**

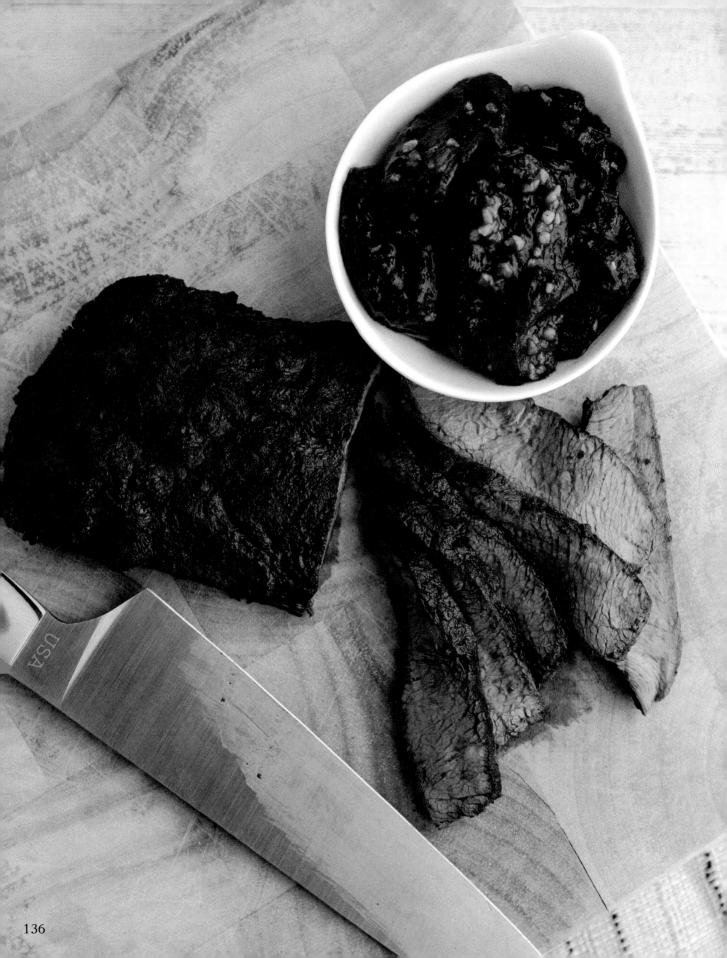

CHIPOTLE FLAT IRON

GRILLED FLAT IRON WITH A SWEET AND SPICY KICK

While the chilies in this ready-made marinade pack quite a bit of heat on their own, the final flavors absorbed into the steak aren't overwhelmingly spicy…instead, adding just enough of a kick. This slightly sweet and savory flat iron goes great sliced alongside a serving of Broiled Green Beans, recipe page: 179.

SHOPPING LIST

1 thin flat iron steak (about 12 ounces)

1 (7-ounce) can chipotles in adobo sauce

2 teaspoons minced garlic

HELPFUL TIPS

This recipe makes enough marinade to marinate two flat iron steaks at the same time if you would like to prepare 4 servings, rather than 2.

1 PLACE flat iron steak in a food storage container or square baking dish.

2 TOP steak with chipotles, adobo sauce from the can, and minced garlic. Flip to coat steak on both sides.

3 COVER and refrigerate steak for 30 minutes, to marinate.

4 OIL a grill or grill pan and preheat on high heat.

5 FLIP steak in marinade to thickly coat before placing on the grill. Discard marinade.

6 GRILL for 5 minutes on each side for medium-rare, just until a meat thermometer registers 145°F.

7 LET rest for at least 5 minutes before thinly slicing against the grain to serve.

MEATS

WHAT MAKES IT QUICK & EASY: The acid and heat of the chipotle peppers allows you to tenderize and marinate this steak in only 30 minutes.

Calories: 435 · Fat: 21g · Protein: 53g · Total Carbs: 4.5g − Fiber: 2.5g = **Net Carbs: 2g**

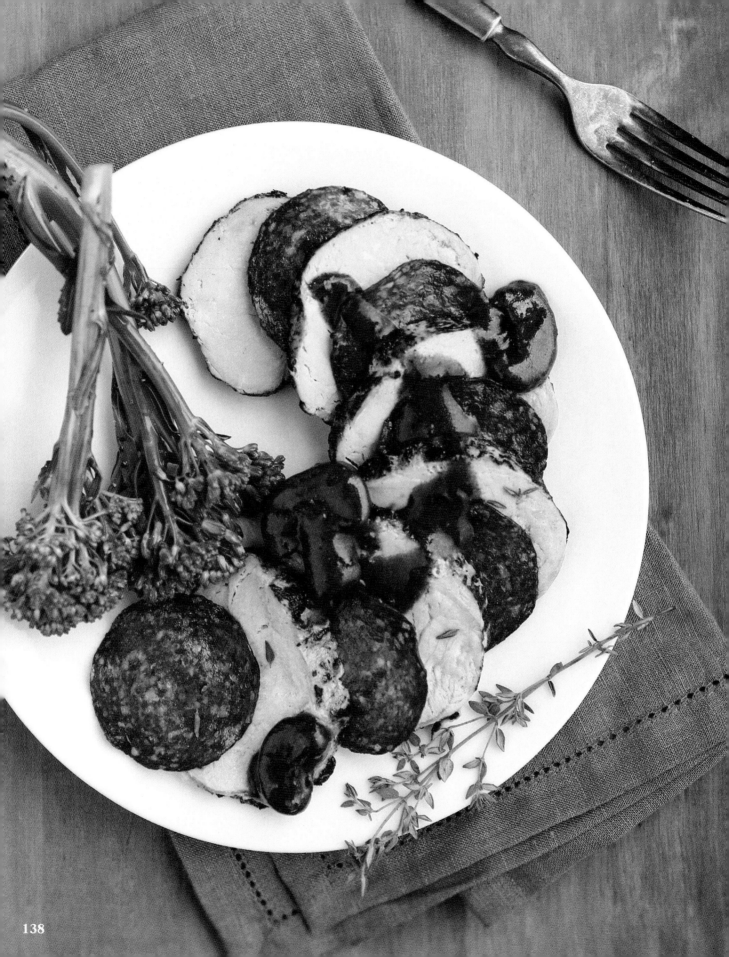

ROASTED PORK WITH CRISPY SALAMI
WITH OR WITHOUT SAVORY BALSAMIC MUSHROOMS

Crispy baked salami is layered in between tender and juicy pork tenderloin in this elegant, yet dead simple dish. I like to serve it topped with my Savory Balsamic Mushrooms, recipe page: 181, but it can also be served alone to save on time. (Nutritional information does not include the Savory Balsamic Mushrooms.)

SHOPPING LIST

1 large pork tenderloin
(about 1¼ pounds)

1 tablespoon olive oil

½ teaspoon dried thyme

½ teaspoon salt

½ teaspoon black pepper

¼ teaspoon garlic powder

12 thin slices genoa salami

1 batch Savory Balsamic Mushrooms, recipe page: 181, if desired

HELPFUL TIPS

This is also great when topped with my Gorgonzola & Chive Butter, recipe page 127.

1 PREHEAT oven to 400°F. Heat the olive oil in a large skillet over high heat.

2 RUB the thyme, salt, pepper, and garlic powder into the pork tenderloin.

3 PLACE the seasoned tenderloin in the hot skillet and brown on all sides.

4 TRANSFER tenderloin to the oven, and bake for 20–24 minutes, or until a meat thermometer inserted into the thickest part registers 145°F.

5 MEANWHILE, line a sheet pan with parchment paper and arrange slices of genoa salami on pan without overlapping.

6 BAKE salami alongside the tenderloin (on any rack) for 10–14 minutes, until crisp.

7 LET pork rest for 10 minutes before slicing thin. Serve by alternating slices of pork with slices of crispy salami. Prepare and top with Savory Balsamic Mushrooms, if desired.

MEATS

WHAT MAKES IT QUICK & EASY: Pork tenderloin is one of the quickest cuts of meat that you can roast.

Calories: 340 • Fat: 18g • Protein: 43g • Total Carbs: 0.5g − Fiber: 0g = **Net Carbs: 0.5g**

MOJO MARINATED SKIRT STEAK
GRILLED STEAK IN A CITRUS AND GARLIC MARINADE

Mojo Criollo is a Cuban marinade with orange, lemon, and garlic that is one of my favorite items to keep in my pantry. The citrus in the marinade does a great job at tenderizing a temperamental cut of meat like skirt steak, which can be tough, but only if you overcook it. Marinating the steak first makes it far more forgiving though, even if you don't nail the temperature.

SHOPPING LIST

2 pounds skirt steak

2 cups Mojo Criollo marinade (see tip)

1 tablespoon olive oil

HELPFUL TIPS

Mojo Criollo is sold in large bottles in the Spanish food section of the grocery store. It does contain a few carbs, but almost all of the marinade is discarded before cooking.

MEATS

1 PLACE skirt steak in a food storage container or square baking dish.

2 POUR Mojo and olive oil over the skirt steak and flip to coat on both sides.

3 COVER and refrigerate steak for at least 2 hours, flipping halfway through.

4 OIL a grill or grill pan, and preheat on high heat.

5 REMOVE steak from marinade, and grill for 5 minutes on each side for medium-rare. I do not recommend cooking skirt steak to higher temperatures.

6 LET rest for 10 minutes before thinly slicing against the grain.

WHAT MAKES IT QUICK & EASY: Marinating the skirt steak is the easiest way to ensure that it will come out tender.

Calories: 500 • Fat: 26g • Protein: 60.5g • Total Carbs: 1g – Fiber: 0g = **Net Carbs: 1g**

CHEESESTEAK "MAC"

WITH SLICED RIBEYE, PEPPERS, AND ONIONS

Remember those boxed meals that begged for "help"? This recipe may be reminiscent of those, but also of the filling inside a Philly cheesesteak sandwich. You can't go wrong with this concoction of all your favorite cheesesteak ingredients combined with Mock Mac & Cheese.

SHOPPING LIST

1 batch Stovetop Mock Mac & Cheese, recipe page: 57

2 teaspoons vegetable oil

1 thick-cut boneless ribeye steak, thinly sliced (12–16 ounces)

½ teaspoon baking soda

⅓ cup diced red onion

½ cup diced bell peppers (any color)

HELPFUL TIPS

Tossing the steak in baking soda slightly tenderizes the meat, but more importantly, actually promotes the browning process. This allows you to brown the outside of the steak without overcooking the thin slices.

1 PREPARE the Stovetop Mock Mac & Cheese according to the recipe's directions.

2 MEANWHILE, heat oil in a large skillet over high heat, until nearly smoking hot.

3 Toss sliced ribeye in baking soda before adding to the hot skillet. Sauté until browned, about 3 minutes. Remove from skillet and cover. Drain excess grease from skillet.

4 REDUCE heat to medium-high. Add onion and peppers to the skillet, and sauté for 3 minutes, stirring constantly, until peppers are crisp-tender.

5 ADD the browned ribeye back into the skillet and remove from heat.

6 WHILE the skillet is still hot, but off the heat, pour the finished Mock Mac & Cheese into the skillet, and stir until all is combined.

MEATS

WHAT MAKES IT QUICK & EASY: This is a quick way to turn my Stovetop Mock Mac & Cheese into a full dinner for the whole family.

Calories: 600 · Fat: 48g · Protein: 36g · Total Carbs: 8.5g − Fiber: 3.5g = **Net Carbs: 5g**

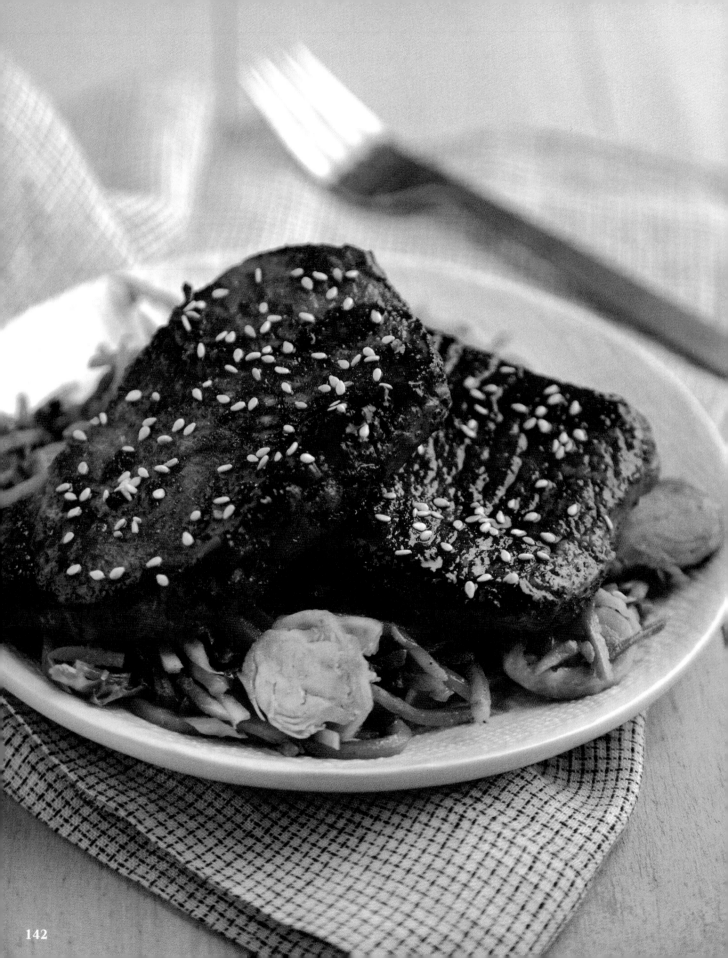

SOY GLAZED PORK CHOPS

BONELESS PORK LOIN CHOPS WITH A SAVORY-SWEET GLAZE

These Asian-style pork chops are a perfect balance of sweet and salty, so it's guaranteed to light up your taste buds. High heat creates a glaze without the need for sugar, and they're made from start to finish in only fifteen minutes!

SHOPPING LIST

1 tablespoon vegetable oil

8 boneless pork loin chops

¼ cup reduced-sodium soy sauce

2½ teaspoons sugar substitute

1 teaspoon minced garlic

¼ teaspoon onion powder

Toasted sesame seeds, for garnish, if desired

HELPFUL TIPS

The glaze in this recipe will eventually begin to stick to the bottom of the pan. This is completely normal, and how you get the most concentrated flavor on the pork by rubbing into the glaze to coat.

1 HEAT oil in a large skillet over medium-high heat, until nearly smoking hot.

2 ADD the pork chops to the hot skillet, and brown well, about 4 minutes on each side.

3 MEANWHILE, in a small bowl, whisk together all remaining ingredients, except sesame seeds, to make the glaze.

4 REDUCE heat to medium and pour the glaze into the skillet. Flip pork chops in the glaze as it bubbles up, reduces, and begins to caramelize.

5 CUT into the thickest chop to reveal that it is mostly white throughout before serving sprinkled with toasted sesame seeds.

MEATS

WHAT MAKES IT QUICK & EASY: By deglazing the pan with soy sauce, this recipe is packed with flavor, without having to marinate the chops beforehand.

Calories: 290 • Fat: 11g • Protein: 46g • Total Carbs: 2g – Fiber: 0g = **Net Carbs: 2g**

JAPANESE SIRLOIN STIR-FRY
WITH ZUCCHINI AND YELLOW ONION

Asian-inspired dishes are always a welcome change when considering the vast variety of ingredients that can be used. Fresh is always best, especially on low-carb, making a stir-fry the perfect dinner option for any night of the week.

SHOPPING LIST

1 tablespoon vegetable oil

1 pound top sirloin, thinly sliced

½ teaspoon baking soda

2 medium zucchini, chopped

½ cup chopped yellow onion

3 tablespoons soy sauce

2 teaspoons rice wine vinegar (may use cider vinegar)

¼ teaspoon black pepper

2 teaspoons sesame oil

MEATS

1 HEAT oil in a large skillet or wok over high heat, until nearly smoking hot.

2 Toss sliced sirloin in baking soda before adding to the hot skillet. Sauté until browned, about 3 minutes. Remove from skillet and cover.

3 REDUCE heat to medium-high. Add all remaining ingredients, except sesame oil, to the skillet, and sauté for 4 minutes, stirring constantly, until zucchini is crisp-tender.

4 STIR the browned sirloin back into the skillet, and add the sesame oil before serving.

HELPFUL TIPS

Tossing the steak in baking soda slightly tenderizes the meat, but more importantly, actually promotes the browning process. This allows you to brown the outside of the steak without overcooking the thin slices.

WHAT MAKES IT QUICK & EASY: Stir-fry, especially on low-carb, is always a quick & easy dinner option!

Calories: 310 · Fat: 15g · Protein: 36.5g · Total Carbs: 5.5g − Fiber: 1.5g = **Net Carbs: 4g**

CHEESEBURGER MEATLOAF

WITH PICKLES, ONIONS, CHEDDAR CHEESE, AND CONDIMENTS

Drive-thrus are a thing of the past for my family, but that doesn't stop us from craving a juicy cheeseburger every now and again. Such a craving hit me one day when my wife Rachel was busy preparing our weekly meatloaf, and I decided "burger-ize" that loaf, condiments and all. It seemed crazy, but the results were delicious. We serve this alongside my Cauliflower Mash, recipe page: 172.

SHOPPING LIST

Nonstick cooking spray

MEATLOAF

2 pounds lean ground beef

1 cup shredded Cheddar cheese

2 large eggs, beaten

¼ cup grated Parmesan cheese

¼ cup minced yellow onion

½ teaspoon onion powder

¾ teaspoon salt

¾ teaspoon black pepper

TOPPING

¼ cup no-sugar added ketchup

1 tablespoon yellow mustard

1 dill pickle, thinly sliced

1 PREHEAT oven to 350°F. Spray a 9x5-inch loaf pan with nonstick cooking spray.

2 IN a large mixing bowl, use your hands to combine all Meatloaf ingredients.

3 TRANSFER the meatloaf mixture to the prepared baking dish and use your hands to form an even top.

4 BAKE for 40 minutes.

5 MEANWHILE, whisk together ketchup and mustard to create the Topping. Top meatloaf with the pickle slices and spread the ketchup Topping over top all.

6 BAKE for 20 additional minutes, or until a meat thermometer inserted into the loaf registers 155°F. Let rest at least 5 minutes before slicing.

HELPFUL TIPS

I like to use lean ground beef in a meatloaf like this, as regular ground beef ends up filling the loaf pan with grease.

WHAT MAKES IT QUICK & EASY: This can be prepared in advance, refrigerated, and baked whenever ready for a fresh meal after a long day.

Calories: 355 • Fat: 20g • Protein: 39.5g • Total Carbs: 2g – Fiber: 0g = **Net Carbs: 2g**

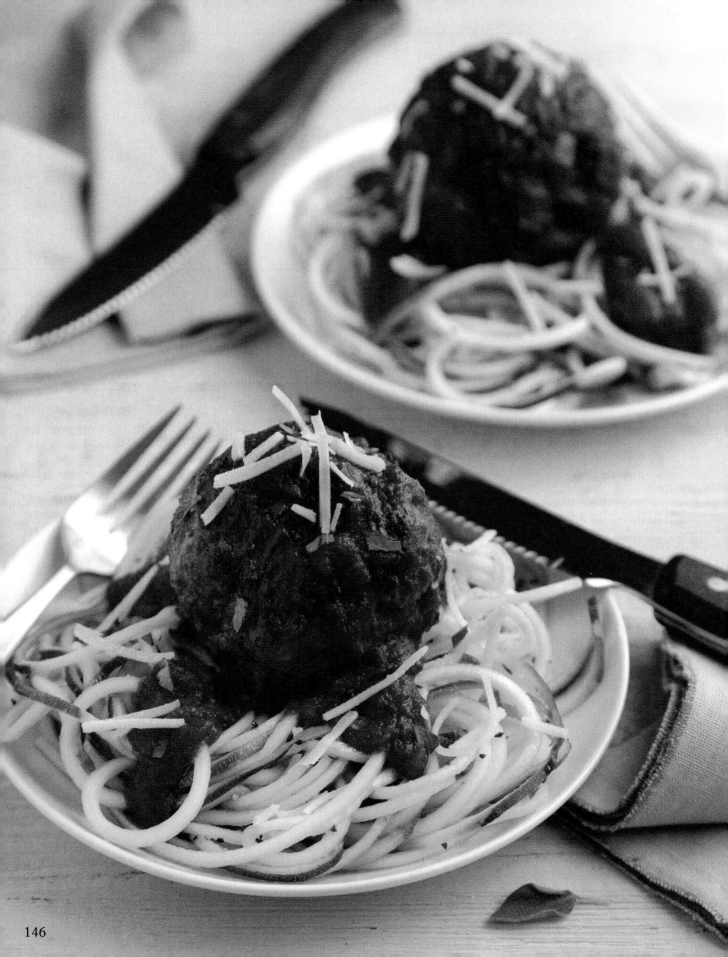

FORK & KNIFE MEATBALLS

GIANT QUARTER-POUND ITALIAN MEATBALLS

You're definitely going to need a fork and knife to tackle these massive meatballs! Parmesan cheese is baked right in to replace breadcrumbs and add more Italian flavor. For a complete and satisfying meal, serve these atop any of my Pasta Alternatives, recipe page: 170.

SHOPPING LIST

Nonstick cooking spray

1 pound ground beef

1 large egg, beaten

⅓ cup grated Parmesan cheese

1 teaspoon Italian seasoning

¾ teaspoon garlic powder

¾ teaspoon salt

¾ teaspoon black pepper

Pasta sauce, if desired, to serve

HELPFUL TIPS

To make this even easier, with softer meatballs, you can skip the browning, and simply bake for 30–35 minutes before tossing in pasta sauce to serve.

1 PREHEAT oven to 350°F. Spray an oven-safe skillet with nonstick cooking spray.

2 COMBINE ground beef and all remaining ingredients, except pasta sauce, in a large mixing bowl.

3 USE your hands to mix and then tightly form the ground beef mixture into 4 giant meatballs.

4 PLACE meatballs in the greased skillet over medium-high heat. Brown well on all sides.

5 TRANSFER skillet to the oven and bake meatballs 20–25 minutes, flipping halfway through. Meatballs are done when a meat thermometer inserted into the center registers 155°F.

6 Toss in pasta sauce before serving, if desired.

MEATS

WHAT MAKES IT QUICK & EASY: With this recipe, you only have to roll 4 meatballs, rather than 16 or more small meatballs.

Calories: 350 • Fat: 21.5g • Protein: 37g • Total Carbs: 0.5g − Fiber: 0g = **Net Carbs: 0.5g**

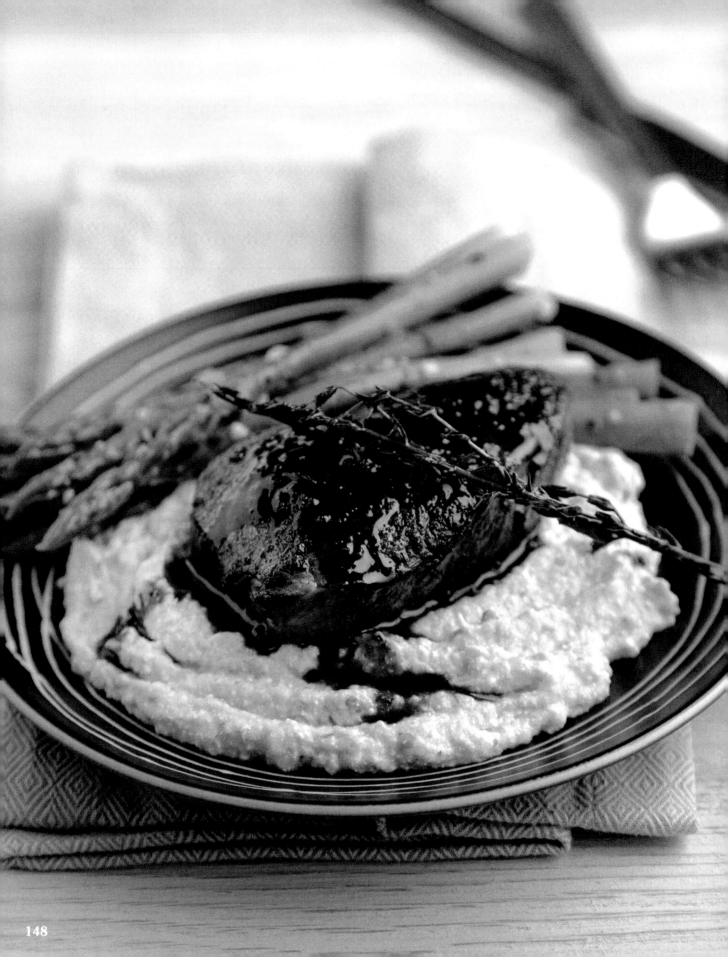

SIRLOIN FILET BALSAMICO

FINE DINING IN A FLASH

It's a common misconception that to get a top quality meal, one must dine out, paying an exorbitant amount of money. That is certainly not the case when you've got a good pan, a good cut of beef, and a plan. Though I rate this filet five stars on its own, it's even better when served over the top of my Creamy Eggplant "Polenta," recipe page: 183.

SHOPPING LIST

2 teaspoons olive oil

2 top sirloin filets (6–8 ounces each)

Salt and black pepper

Garlic powder

2 sprigs fresh thyme

2 tablespoons balsamic vinegar

1 teaspoon sugar substitute

2 tablespoons unsalted butter

HELPFUL TIPS

Be sure to use ordinary balsamic vinegar in this recipe and not "balsamic glaze," as glaze has already been reduced with tons of added sugar. Flavored balsamic vinegars are also great, as long as they have no added sugar.

1 HEAT oil in a large skillet over medium-high heat, until nearly smoking hot.

2 GENEROUSLY season sirloin filets with salt, pepper, and garlic powder before adding to the hot skillet. Top each steak with a sprig of fresh thyme.

3 BROWN steaks well, about 5 minutes on each side. For medium-rare, a meat thermometer stuck into the thickest steak should read about 135°F at this stage of cooking.

4 MEANWHILE, in a small bowl, whisk together balsamic vinegar and sugar substitute to make the glaze.

5 REDUCE heat to medium and pour the glaze into the skillet. Flip steaks in the glaze as it bubbles up, reduces, and begins to caramelize.

6 REMOVE skillet from heat and stir butter into the glaze to thicken. Let steaks rest at least 5 minutes before serving drizzled with the glaze.

MEATS

WHAT MAKES IT QUICK & EASY: You'd usually be hard pressed to make an entrée this elegant in this little time.

Calories: 505 • Fat: 40g • Protein: 33g • Total Carbs: 0.5g − Fiber: 0g = **Net Carbs: 0.5g**

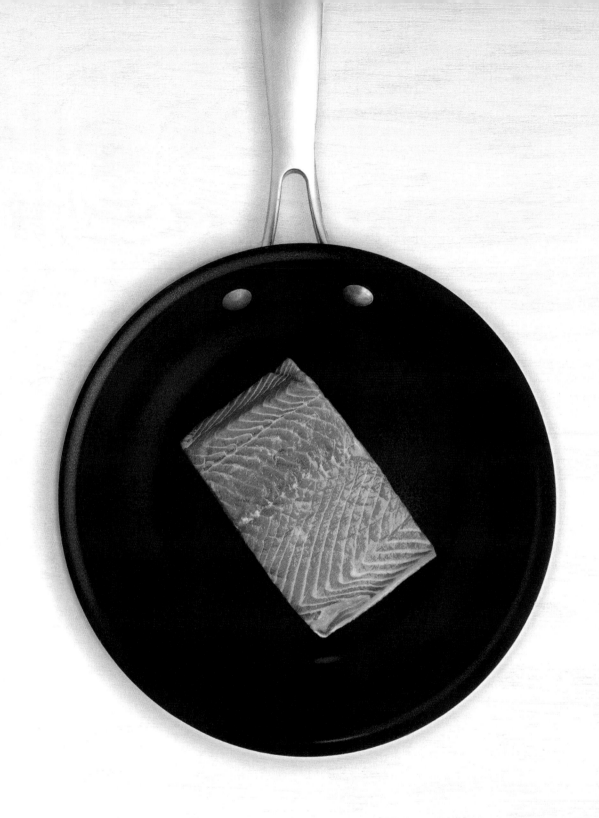

SEAFOOD

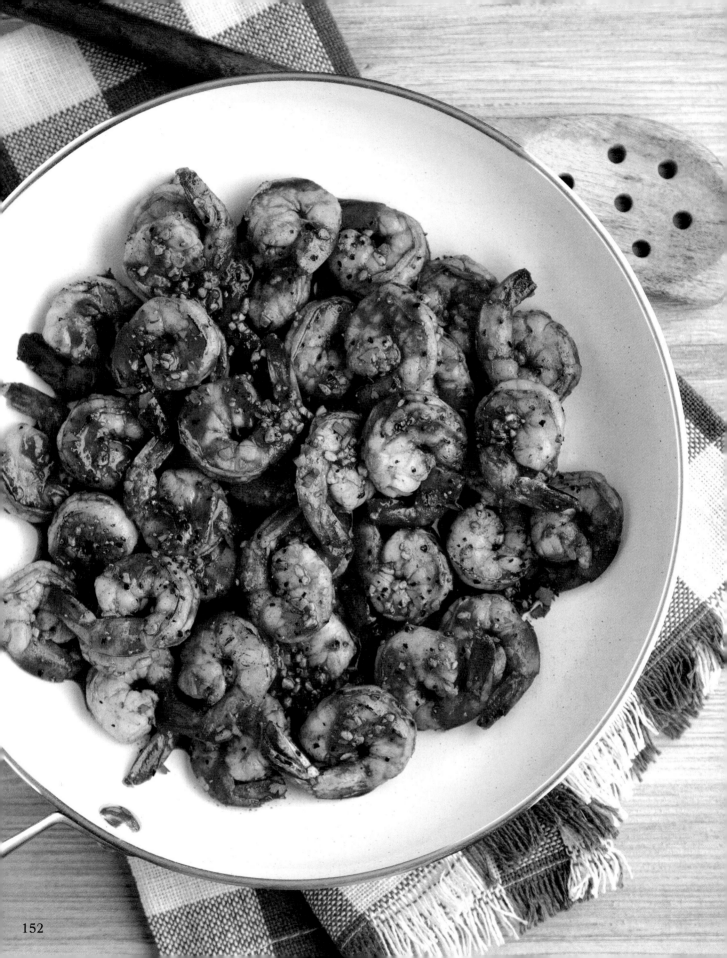

SMOKED PAPRIKA SHRIMP
SMOKEY AND SWEET SAUTÉED SHRIMP

The sweet smokiness and rich color of this shrimp sauté is as pleasing to the eyes as it is to the palate— something that could only be achieved by smoked paprika. These shrimp may not even make it to your plate, which is fine, because I've been known to eat them straight out of the pan.

SHOPPING LIST

1 pound large peeled shrimp, tail-on, if desired

1 tablespoon olive oil

2 teaspoons smoked paprika

2 teaspoons minced garlic

¼ teaspoon salt

¼ teaspoon black pepper

Juice of ½ lemon

1 tablespoon unsalted butter

Chopped parsley, for garnish

HELPFUL TIPS

Smoked paprika is now easily found in the spice aisle of the grocery store (it used to be much harder to find). It's now an indispensable ingredient for me!

1 HEAT a skillet over medium-high heat.

2 IN a mixing bowl, toss shrimp with olive oil, smoked paprika, garlic, salt, and pepper.

3 ADD seasoned shrimp to the hot skillet, and sauté for 2 minutes, just until they begin to brown.

4 SQUEEZE lemon juice over the shrimp, and sauté 1 additional minute, just until shrimp are opaque in the center.

5 REMOVE from heat and stir in butter. Sprinkle with chopped parsley, if desired, before serving.

SEAFOOD

WHAT MAKES IT QUICK & EASY: With a 3-minute cook time, you don't get much quicker than sautéed shrimp!

Calories: 150 • Fat: 6.5g • Protein: 21.5g • Total Carbs: 3g – Fiber: 0g = **Net Carbs: 3g**

TILAPIA WITH MELON SALSA
SPICED TILIAPIA WITH COOLING SALSA

If you're not into spicy food, don't count this seared tilapia out quite yet. The cool sweetness of honeydew melon balances nicely with the spiced fish, cooling off some of the heat. There is a lot to love about the complexity of this dish, especially when considering it'll be prepped and done in only twenty minutes.

SHOPPING LIST

1 tablespoon olive oil

2 tilapia fillets

½ teaspoon chili powder

¼ teaspoon ground cumin

¼ teaspoon salt

¼ teaspoon black pepper

1 pinch ground cayenne pepper

MELON SALSA

½ cup diced honeydew melon

Juice of ½ lemon

2 tablespoons diced red onion

1 tablespoon chopped fresh cilantro

Salt and black pepper

1 HEAT the olive oil in a large sauté pan over medium-high heat, until nearly smoking hot.

2 SEASON the tilapia with chili powder, cumin, salt, pepper, and cayenne, and place into the hot pan. Let sear for 3 minutes without moving the fish.

3 FLIP tilapia, and let cook for 2 additional minutes, or until fish is flaky.

4 MEANWHILE, in a small mixing bowl, toss together all Melon Salsa ingredients, seasoning with salt and pepper to taste.

5 SERVE each tilapia fillet topped with ½ of the Melon Salsa.

HELPFUL TIPS

Buying a small container of honeydew melon chunks will save you from having to buy and cut a whole melon just to make the salsa in this recipe.

WHAT MAKES IT QUICK & EASY: Like most seafood, tilapia only takes minutes to cook!

Calories: 225 • Fat: 8.5g • Protein: 32g • Total Carbs: 6.5g − Fiber: 0.5g = **Net Carbs: 6g**

SEAFOOD

ROSEMARY ROASTED HALIBUT
WITH ORANGE ZEST

This oven roasted flatfish dish could make planning a date night all too easy. The combination of ingredients offers a touch of elegance without much fuss, leaving you more time to spend with that special someone.

SHOPPING LIST

1 pound halibut, cut into 2 fillets

1 tablespoon olive oil

½ teaspoon paprika

¼ teaspoon salt

¼ teaspoon black pepper

2 teaspoons orange zest

2 large sprigs rosemary

Lemon wedges, to serve

HELPFUL TIPS

You can also make this with lemon zest in place of the orange zest to simplify your shopping list; however, the orange goes great with the rosemary.

1 PREHEAT oven to 450°F. Line a sheet pan with parchment paper.

2 Toss halibut fillets in olive oil, paprika, salt, and pepper, making sure the fish is oiled on all sides.

3 PLACE fillets on the prepared sheet pan and sprinkle orange zest over the top of each. Top each fillet with a sprig of rosemary.

4 BAKE for 10 minutes, or until flaking with a fork reveals that they are opaque throughout. Serve with lemon wedges for squeezing over top.

WHAT MAKES IT QUICK & EASY: The prep of this recipe takes so little time that you're sure to have it finished before the oven has even preheated.

Calories: 300 • Fat: 12g • Protein: 47g • Total Carbs: 1g – Fiber: 0g = **Net Carbs: 1g**

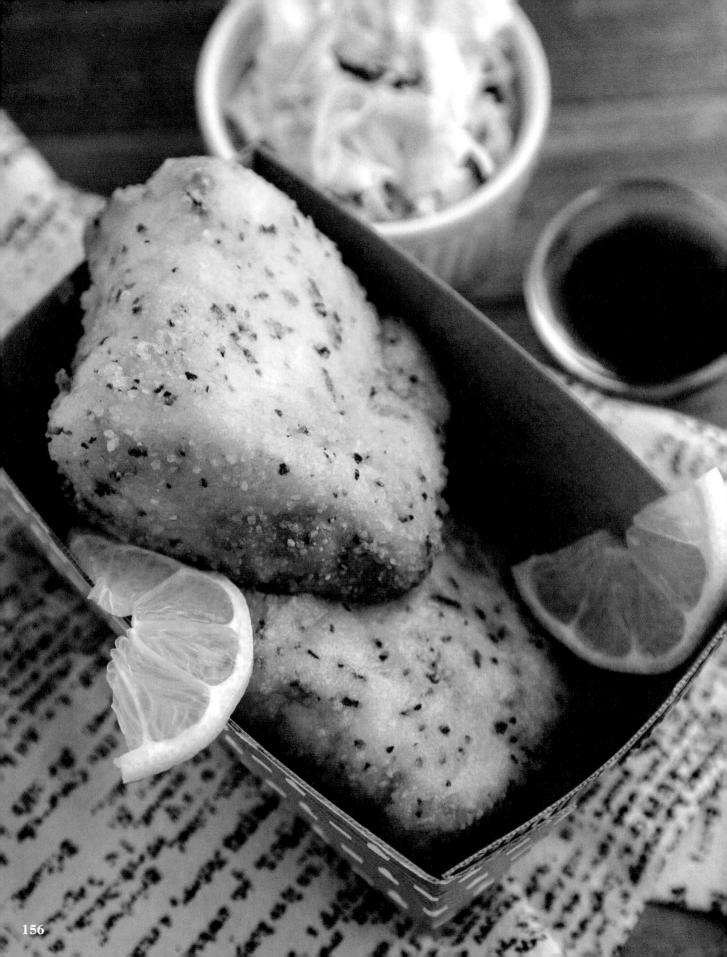

FRIED COD

WITH LEMON ZEST AND BLACK PEPPER BREADING

Cod battered and fried without the use of a single breadcrumb, you ask? Yes, that's right. Parmesan cheese makes a perfect breading that crisps up just as the fish is cooked throughout.

SHOPPING LIST

2 large eggs

¼ teaspoon salt

1 cup grated Parmesan cheese

Zest of 1 lemon

¾ teaspoon black pepper

4 small or 2 large cod fillets

Vegetable oil, for shallow frying

HELPFUL TIPS

Frozen cod fillets can be used to prepare this, but they should be fully thawed in the fridge, and dried of excess water, using paper towels before breading.

1 IN a shallow but wide bowl, whisk eggs with salt to create an egg wash.

2 IN a separate bowl, combine Parmesan cheese, lemon zest, and pepper to create a breading.

3 DIP cod fillets in the egg wash, flipping to thoroughly coat. Transfer to the breading mixture, and press the fish into the cheese to ensure the breading adheres.

4 FILL a large skillet with about ¾-inch of vegetable oil, and place over medium-high heat. Let the oil heat up for about 2 minutes.

5 PLACE the breaded cod in the skillet, and cook until golden brown, about 3 minutes on each side. Do this in two batches, if your skillet is too small.

6 TRANSFER fish to paper towels to drain, and check the thickest fillet to ensure it easily flakes with a fork. If the fish is still tough and translucent, return to the oil for 1 additional minute on each side.

7 SERVE immediately with lemon wedges, malt vinegar, or both.

SEAFOOD

WHAT MAKES IT QUICK & EASY: You'd be hard pressed to drive to a fried fish drive-thru in the time it takes to make this recipe.

Calories: 440 · Fat: 27g · Protein: 48.5g · Total Carbs: 0.5g − Fiber: 0g = **Net Carbs: 0.5g**

BACON UNWRAPPED SCALLOPS
A CLASSIC COMBINATION, MADE FOOLPROOF

While these scallops aren't wrapped as you'd expect, the bacon is still there, and that's all that really matters. By leaving things "Unwrapped," you ensure that the bacon is crisp, and the scallops are perfectly cooked, for perfect results every time.

SHOPPING LIST

4 strips thick-sliced bacon, chopped

1¼ pounds sea scallops, patted dry

¼ cup diced yellow onion

1½ teaspoons minced garlic

¼ teaspoon black pepper

Juice of ½ lemon

1 tablespoon chopped fresh parsley

HELPFUL TIPS

Use a slotted spoon when serving, that way you can drain any excess bacon grease. But on the flip side, you may want to drizzle a small amount of that grease over top of the scallops after plating to keep them moist and flavorful.

SEAFOOD

1 COOK chopped bacon in a large skillet over medium-high heat, until nearly crisp.

2 ADD scallops, yellow onion, garlic, and pepper to the skillet, and let scallops cook for 2 minutes without moving them.

3 FLIP scallops, and squeeze lemon juice over top of all. Let cook for an additional 1½ minutes, and cook for an additional 1½ minutes on the opposite side, or until lightly browned.

4 SPRINKLE parsley over top of all before serving.

WHAT MAKES IT QUICK & EASY: In traditional bacon-wrapped scallops, it's very hard to get the bacon crisp without overcooking the scallops.

Calories: 195 • Fat: 7g • Protein: 27g • Total Carbs: 4.5g − Fiber: 0g = **Net Carbs: 4.5g**

FIVE-SPICE SALMON

PAN-SEARED SALMON WITH ASIAN SPICES

Your taste buds are sure to be swimming after the first bite of these salmon fillets. The complexity of the spices used might even fool you into believing your taste buds swam all the way to another continent.

SHOPPING LIST

2 tablespoons vegetable oil

4 (6-ounce) salmon fillets

2 teaspoons five-spice powder

¼ teaspoon salt

2 teaspoons rice wine vinegar

1 tablespoon chopped fresh fennel fronds, optional

HELPFUL TIPS

The fennel fronds add a bright and fresh flavor that pairs with the five-spice, as fennel is one of those five spices. However, you can skip them if you cannot find fresh fennel.

1 HEAT oil in a large skillet over medium-high heat.

2 SEASON salmon fillets with five-spice powder and salt.

3 ADD salmon to the hot skillet and let cook, without moving, until the sides begin to brown and raise up from the pan, about 3 minutes. If using skin-on salmon, add to the pan skin-side down to brown the skin first.

4 FLIP salmon fillets, drizzle with rice wine vinegar, and top with chopped fennel.

5 COVER pan, reduce heat to medium, and let cook an additional 3 minutes.

6 USE a fork to check for doneness. Fish should flake at the edges, but still be cooked medium in the center. Serve immediately.

SEAFOOD

WHAT MAKES IT QUICK & EASY: This is fresh-cooked seafood prepped and cooked in only 12 minutes!

Calories: 290 • Fat: 17g • Protein: 33g • Total Carbs: 1g – Fiber: 0g = **Net Carbs: 1g**

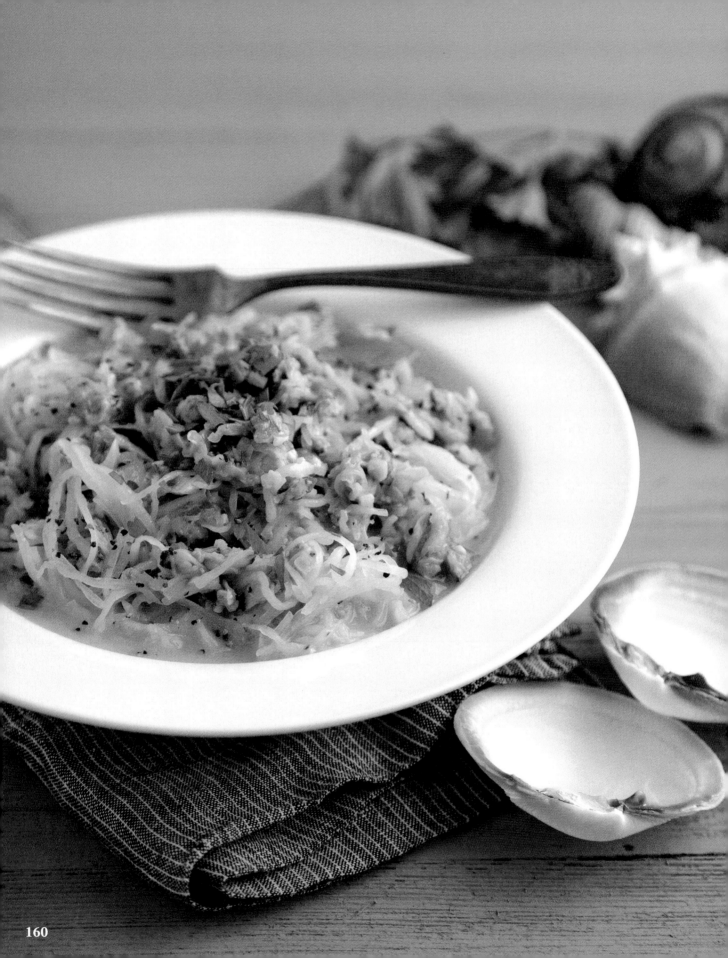

SPAGHETTI SQUASH WITH CLAM SAUCE
CLASSIC CLAM SAUCE, WITHOUT THE HASSLE

Canned clams may not sound like an ingredient a chef would use, but I assure you that we do. In fact, in a recipe for clam sauce like this one, they couldn't be more perfect, as they come with the clam broth needed to develop a deeper flavor.

SHOPPING LIST

2 teaspoons olive oil

2 (10-ounce) cans whole baby clams

2 tablespoons minced red onion

1 tablespoon minced garlic

¼ cup dry white wine (see tip)

1 batch Spaghetti Squash, recipe page: 170

3 tablespoons unsalted butter

2 tablespoons chopped fresh parsley

Salt and black pepper

HELPFUL TIPS

If you'd like to prepare this without white wine, you may use the juice of ½ lemon and a pinch of sugar substitute to replicate the acid and sweetness.

1 HEAT vegetable oil in a large skillet over medium-high heat.

2 DRAIN both cans of clams, reserving the liquid of only 1 can.

3 PLACE red onion and garlic in the skillet, and sauté 1 minute, just until fragrant.

4 ADD white wine and the reserved juice of 1 can of clams to the skillet, and bring up to a boil. Boil until liquid has reduced by about half.

5 ADD the clams and Spaghetti Squash to the liquid in the skillet, and toss to fully coat. Cook just 1 minute to heat the clams.

6 REMOVE from heat, and stir in butter and parsley. Season with salt and pepper to taste before serving.

SEAFOOD

WHAT MAKES IT QUICK & EASY: By using canned clams, you not only save money, but you don't have to scrub the shells and remove the clams from them.

Calories: 205 • Fat: 11.5g • Protein: 15g • Total Carbs: 9g – Fiber: 1.5g = **Net Carbs: 7.5g**

EASY GREEK SHRIMP

WITH MY KALAMATA OLIVE COMPOUND BUTTER

It doesn't get any easier than tossing a few fresh ingredients into a skillet, and within mere minutes, calling dinner done. The Greek flavors in this recipe come largely from my Kalamata Olive Butter, recipe page: 127, which can be prepared several days or even weeks in advance (and stored in the freezer).

SHOPPING LIST

4 tablespoons Kalamata Olive Butter, recipe page: 127, divided

1 pound large shrimp

1 tomato, diced

Chopped oregano, for garnish

HELPFUL TIPS

You can prepare this dish using frozen shrimp by first placing the shrimp in a colander and running cold water over them for 5 minutes, to thaw. They will likely still be very cold in the center, so you should expect that they will take an additional minute to sauté.

1 HEAT 2 tablespoons of the Kalamata Olive butter in a skillet over medium-high heat, until sizzling.

2 ADD shrimp to the hot skillet, and sauté for 3 minutes, just until they are opaque in the center.

3 REMOVE from heat, and stir in diced tomato and the remaining 2 tablespoons of Kalamata Olive butter. Sprinkle with chopped oregano, if desired, before serving.

SEAFOOD

WHAT MAKES IT QUICK & EASY: When you have my Kalamata Olive Butter in your freezer, you're always ready to prepare this dish in mere minutes.

Calories: 185 • Fat: 9.5g • Protein: 21.5g • Total Carbs: 3.5g − Fiber: 0g = **Net Carbs: 3.5g**

TILAPIA WITH BASIL & CAPERS

TOPPED WITH A QUICK BUTTER SAUCE

This light and buttery entrée gives new meaning to "quick and easy." In only fifteen minutes, you'll end up with a dish similar to what you might find listed on a menu somewhere along the coastline of the Mediterranean.

SHOPPING LIST

2 teaspoons olive oil

2 tilapia fillets

Salt and black pepper

2 teaspoons minced garlic

Juice of ½ lemon

2 tablespoons sliced basil

2 tablespoons capers, drained

2 tablespoons unsalted butter

HELPFUL TIPS

This can also be made with cod or other white fish fillets.

1 HEAT the olive oil in a large sauté pan over medium-high heat, until nearly smoking hot.

2 SEASON the tilapia with salt and pepper, and place into the hot pan. Let sear for 3 minutes without moving the fish.

3 FLIP tilapia, add garlic to the pan in the empty spaces between the fillets, and squeeze lemon over top of all.

4 LET cook for 2 additional minutes, or until fish is flaky. Transfer fish to serving plates.

5 REMOVE pan from heat, and add basil, capers, and butter, stirring to mix with juices from the pan. Drizzle over top of each serving of tilapia.

SEAFOOD

WHAT MAKES IT QUICK & EASY: Because it is so popular, tilapia is one of the easiest fish to find fresh at the grocery store.

Calories: 295 • Fat: 18g • Protein: 32g • Total Carbs: 3g − Fiber: 0g = **Net Carbs: 3g**

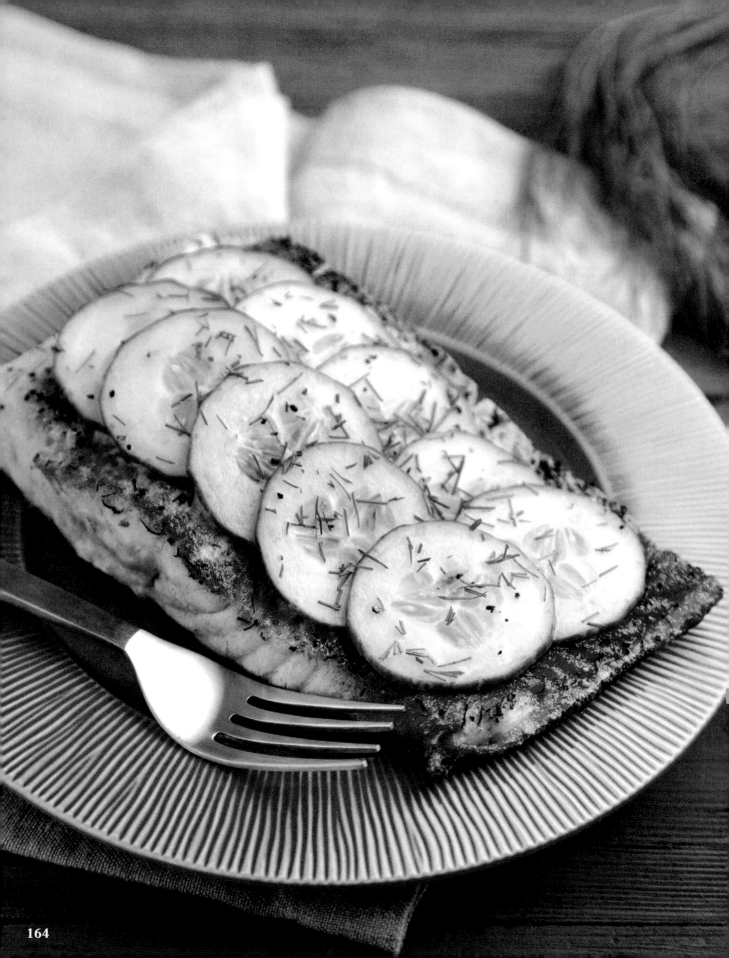

SALMON WITH CUCUMBER & DILL

LIGHTLY PICKLED CUCUMBER TOPPED SALMON

Don't be deceived by the sophisticated appearance of this dish. While the results are beautiful, it is quite simple to prepare and tastes even better than it looks. The sliced cucumber actually pickles while the salmon cooks, adding a nice crispness that pairs perfectly without overpowering the fish.

SHOPPING LIST

PICKLED CUCUMBER

1 cucumber, very thinly sliced

1 tablespoon cider vinegar

2 teaspoons chopped fresh dill

1 teaspoon sugar substitute

¼ teaspoon salt

¼ teaspoon black pepper

SALMON

2 tablespoons vegetable oil, divided

4 (6-ounce) salmon fillets

2 teaspoons cider vinegar

1 tablespoon chopped fresh dill

¼ teaspoon salt

¼ teaspoon black pepper

HELPFUL TIPS

I find English cucumbers look better than regular cucumbers when topping the salmon, however, either will work. You'll only need to use ½ of an English cucumber as they are much longer.

1 IN a mixing bowl, toss together all Pickled Cucumber ingredients, and let marinate as you cook the salmon.

2 HEAT 1 tablespoon of the vegetable oil in a large skillet over medium-high heat.

3 IN a clean mixing bowl, toss salmon fillets with the remaining tablespoon of vegetable oil and all remaining salmon ingredients, until well coated.

4 ADD coated salmon to the hot skillet and let cook, without moving, until the sides begin to brown, and raise up from the pan, about 3 minutes. If using skin-on salmon, add to the pan skin-side down to brown the skin first.

5 FLIP salmon fillets, cover pan, reduce heat to medium, and let cook an additional 3 minutes.

6 USE a fork to check for doneness. Fish should flake at the edges, but still be cooked medium in the center.

7 TRANSFER fillets to serving plates. Arrange a thin layer of Pickled Cucumber over top each salmon fillet before serving.

SEAFOOD

WHAT MAKES IT QUICK & EASY: This is a restaurant-quality dish you can have on the table in only about 20 minutes!

Calories: 295 • Fat: 17.5g • Protein: 33.5g • Total Carbs: 2g – Fiber: 0g = **Net Carbs: 2g**

SHORTCUT PESTO COD LOINS

TOPPED WITH FRESH TOMATO

Pesto brightens up this flaky white fish with its characteristic combination of basil, Parmesan cheese, and pine nuts. Diced tomato adds a finishing touch of freshness and color, sprinkled over the top, directly after baking.

SHOPPING LIST

2 cod loins (see tip)

¼ cup prepared pesto sauce

¼ cup diced tomato

1 teaspoon lemon juice

1 pinch pepper

HELPFUL TIPS

Cod loins are the thicker part of the cod fillet, and can more easily stand up to the dry heat of roasting than thin fillets. If you cannot find them fresh, grocery stores will typically have high-quality loins frozen. Simply thaw in the fridge before preparing this recipe.

1 PREHEAT oven to 400°F. Line a sheet pan with parchment paper.

2 PLACE cod loins on the prepared sheet pan, and 2 tablespoons of pesto over each.

3 BAKE for 10–12 minutes, just until flaking with a fork reveals that they are opaque throughout.

4 MEANWHILE, in a small mixing bowl, toss diced tomato with lemon juice and pepper.

5 TOP each cod loin with 2 tablespoons of the tomatoes before serving.

SEAFOOD

WHAT MAKES IT QUICK & EASY: Using prepared pesto sauce (we buy the refrigerated kind) saves not only time, but money, as pine nuts are not cheap!

Calories: 320 • Fat: 15g • Protein: 43.5g • Total Carbs: 3g – Fiber: 0.5g = **Net Carbs: 2.5g**

SCALLOP & BOK CHOY STIR-FRY

SWEET SCALLOPS WITH TENDER CABBAGE

Known to some as "Chinese cabbage," bok choy lends a mellow flavor along with a crisp freshness to this Asian scallop stir-fry. Rice wine vinegar adds acidity, but also a touch of sweetness. Bell pepper adds a touch of red to offset the green bok choy.

SHOPPING LIST

1 tablespoon vegetable oil

1¼ pounds sea scallops, patted dry

8 ounces chopped bok choy

¼ cup diced red bell pepper

2 teaspoons minced garlic

2 tablespoons soy sauce

1 tablespoon rice wine vinegar

½ teaspoon sugar substitute

2 teaspoons sesame oil

HELPFUL TIPS

Bok choy makes the perfect choice in this recipe, as it takes the same amount of time to stir-fry as the scallops.

1 HEAT vegetable oil in a large skillet or wok over medium-high heat.

2 PLACE scallops in the skillet first, then bok choy, bell pepper, and garlic over the top. Let cook for 2 minutes without stirring.

3 ADD soy sauce, vinegar, and sugar substitute to the skillet, and toss to combine. Stir-fry for an additional 2–3 minutes, just until bok choy is crisp-tender, and scallops are opaque in the center.

4 STIR in sesame oil before serving.

SEAFOOD

WHAT MAKES IT QUICK & EASY: As I've said throughout this book, stir-fry is the king of quick and easy meals!

Calories: 190 • Fat: 7g • Protein: 25g • Total Carbs: 6g − Fiber: 0.5g = **Net Carbs: 5.5g**

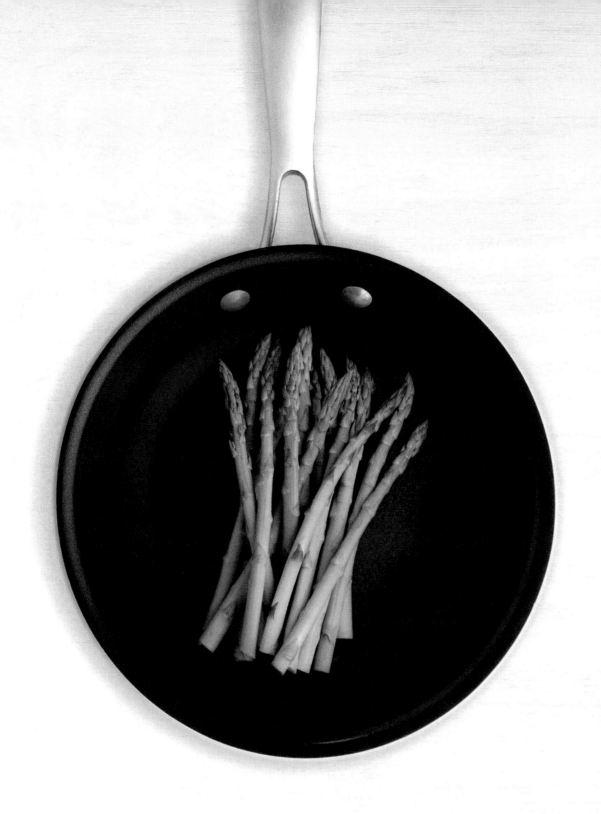

SIDE DISHES

SIDES

QUICK & EASY
PASTA ALTERNATIVES

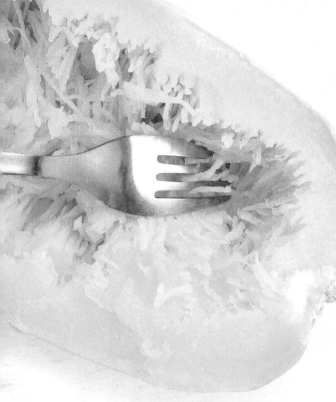

SPAGHETTI SQUASH

4 SERVINGS

1 spaghetti squash, cut in half lengthwise.

1 USING a spoon, scrape seeds and fiberous pulp from the center of each half of the squash. Discard pulp.

2 PIERCE the rind of both halves of the squash in several places with the tip of a sharp knife to help vent the heat as it cooks.

3 PLACE halves, cut side down, on a large plate and microwave on high for 6–8 minutes, just until rind is tender when pierced with a fork.

Calories: 30 • Fat: 0g • Protein: 0.5g
Total Carbs: 6.5g – Fiber: 1.5g = **Net Carbs: 5g**

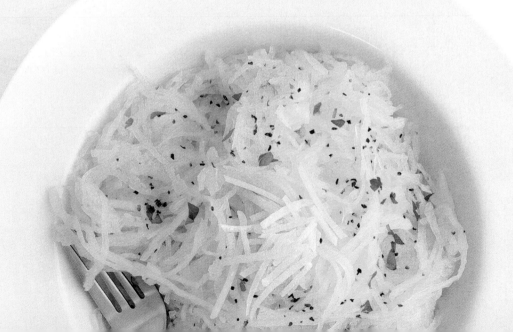

ZUCCHINI NOODLES

1 SERVING PER ZUCCHINI

1 large zucchini

1 TRIM both ends from zucchini and discard.

2 USE the thin-spiral blade of a vegetable spiralizer to create the noodles.

3 DROP zucchini noodles into boiling water and cook for just 1 minute before draining to serve.

Calories: 35 • Fat: 0g • Protein: 2.5g
Total Carbs: 7.5g – Fiber: 2.5g = **Net Carbs: 5g**

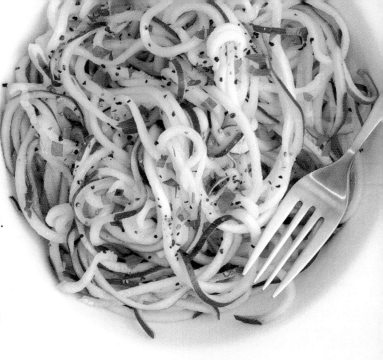

ZUCCHINI RIBBONS

1 SERVING PER ZUCCHINI

1 large zucchini

1 TRIM bottom from zucchini and discard.

2 HOLDING the top of the zucchini, use a vegetable peeler to thinly slice length-wise, into long ribbons. Discard top.

3 DROP zucchini ribbons into boiling water and cook for just 1 minute before draining to serve.

Calories: 35 • Fat: 0g • Protein: 2.5g
Total Carbs: 7.5g – Fiber: 2.5g = **Net Carbs: 5g**

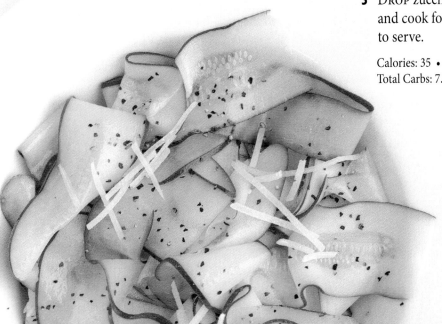

SIDES

QUICK & EASY CAULIFLOWER STAPLES

CAULIFLOWER MASH

4 SERVINGS

1 medium head cauliflower

¼ cup grated Parmesan cheese

2 ounces cream cheese, softened

1 tablespoon unsalted butter, softened

½ teaspoon minced garlic

¼ teaspoon onion powder

¼ teaspoon salt

¼ teaspoon black pepper

1 CUT cauliflower into small pieces, stem and all.

2 ADD chopped cauliflower to boiling water and cook for 6 minutes, or until tender.

3 DRAIN cauliflower very well, but do not cool.

4 ADD drained cauliflower and all remaining ingredients to a food processor and process until smooth. Serve immediately. If cooled, cover and microwave in 15-second intervals until hot.

Calories: 135 • Fat: 10g • Protein: 6.5g
Total Carbs: 6.5g – Fiber: 3g = **Net Carbs: 3.5g**

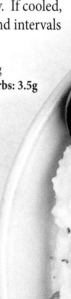

SIDES

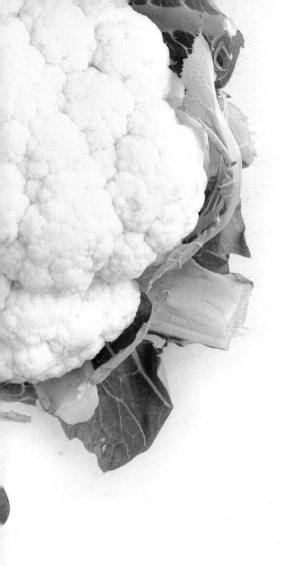

CAULIFLOWER RICE

4 SERVINGS

2 tablespoons unsalted butter

1 (16-ounce) bag cauliflower crumbles
(or 1 small head cauliflower, grated)

3 tablespoons finely diced red onion

1 teaspoon minced garlic

1 teaspoon dry rubbed sage

½ cup chicken stock

1 tablespoon chopped parsley

Salt and black pepper

1 HEAT butter in a nonstick skillet over
medium-high heat, until sizzling.

2 ADD cauliflower, red onion, garlic, and sage to
the skillet and sauté 3 minutes.

3 ADD chicken stock to the skillet and let
simmer 4 minutes, or until cauliflower
is tender.

4 STIR in parsley and season to taste with salt
and pepper before serving.

Calories: 85 • Fat: 6g • Protein: 2.5g
Total Carbs: 7g – Fiber: 3g = **Net Carbs: 4g**

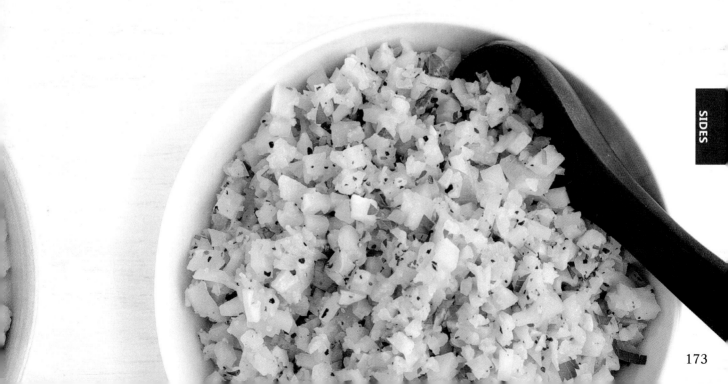

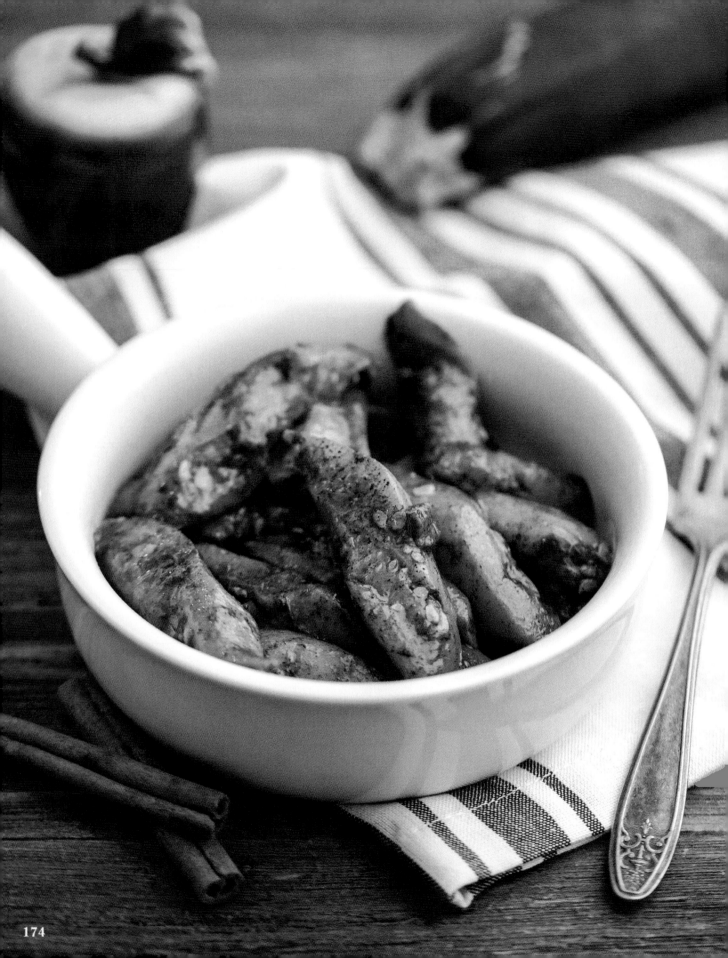

FAUX FRIED APPLES

A LOW-CARB TWIST ON A CLASSIC COUNTRY SIDE DISH

Fried apples are technically a side dish at restaurants such as Cracker Barrel, but they also make for a great dessert, as they are practically just the inside of an apple pie. Reinventing them for low-carb was no small task, but I promise you that I've done it! Using zucchini in place of the apples gives you the right texture, without those pesky carbs. Serve this alongside any pork dish for a great pairing, and then maybe you'll want to serve it again for dessert!

SHOPPING LIST

2 large zucchini

3 tablespoons unsalted butter

¼ cup sugar substitute

½ teaspoon ground cinnamon

¼ teaspoon rum extract (see tip)

¼ teaspoon vanilla extract

HELPFUL TIPS

Additional vanilla extract can be used as a substitution for the rum extract in a pinch.

1 CUT zucchini in half lengthwise, then cut on a bias into 1-inch thick (half-moon) slices.

2 HEAT butter in large skillet over medium-high heat.

3 ADD zucchini to the skillet and sauté 5 minutes, or until lightly browned but still firm.

4 ADD all remaining ingredients to the skillet and sauté for 2 additional minutes, just until zucchini is tender.

5 SERVE hot or cold, as a side or as a dessert. When serving as a dessert, we like to top with sugar-free whipped cream.

WHAT MAKES IT QUICK & EASY: With only a 7-minute cook time, you'll have this on the table before the entrée.

Calories: 105 · Fat: 9g · Protein: 2g · Total Carbs: 6g – Fiber: 2g = **Net Carbs: 4g**

SIDES

MAPLE BACON BRUSSELS SPROUTS
A SWEET AND SAVORY SPROUT SIDE DISH

Bacon and Brussels sprouts were always meant to be together. Add an essence of maple to the mix, and this simple side dish quickly steals the spotlight.

SHOPPING LIST

4 strips thick-cut bacon, diced

1 pound Brussels sprouts, trimmed and halved

¼ cup diced yellow onion

2 teaspoons sugar substitute

1 teaspoon cider vinegar

½ teaspoon maple extract

¼ teaspoon salt

¼ teaspoon black pepper

1 tablespoon unsalted butter

HELPFUL TIPS

If Brussels sprouts begin to get too browned for your liking before they are tender, simply add a splash of water to the pan.

1 SAUTÉ diced bacon in a large skillet over medium-high heat, until crisp. Remove from skillet and set aside. Leave bacon grease in skillet.

2 ADD the Brussels sprouts to the greased skillet. You should be able to hear them sizzling and sauté until they begin to caramelize, about 5 minutes.

3 REDUCE heat to medium-low and stir the yellow onion, sugar substitute, cider vinegar, maple extract, salt, and pepper into the skillet.

4 COVER skillet and let cook for 5 minutes, or until brussels sprouts are crisp-tender.

5 REMOVE from heat and stir in butter and the cooked bacon before serving.

WHAT MAKES IT QUICK & EASY: This recipe gives you all the flavors of roasted Brussels sprouts, without preheating the oven.

Calories: 175 • Fat: 12g • Protein: 7g • Total Carbs: 11g – Fiber: 4.5g = **Net Carbs: 6.5g**

SIDES

BROCCOLI WITH SMOKED GOUDA CREAM SAUCE

A SMOKY TWIST ON BROCCOLI WITH CHEESE SAUCE

When our two kids were younger, my wife Rachel and I found that there was no easier trick to get them to eat their vegetables than by smothering greens with cheese sauce. After all, Cheddar makes everything better, am I right? Well, broccoli has matured a bit, dressed in its new best friend—smoked Gouda!

SHOPPING LIST

16 ounces broccoli florets

½ cup heavy cream

¼ teaspoon garlic powder

¼ teaspoon salt

¼ teaspoon black pepper

4 ounces smoked Gouda cheese, rind removed, diced

HELPFUL TIPS

This can be made even easier by using a bag of ready-to-steam fresh broccoli and microwaving as you measure out the remaining ingredients.

1 BOIL or steam broccoli florets for 4–5 minutes, until crisp-tender. Drain well.

2 TRANSFER drained broccoli to a sauce pot over medium heat and add heavy cream, garlic powder, salt, and pepper.

3 STIRRING frequently, bring the heavy cream in the pot to a simmer. Let simmer for 2 minutes.

4 REMOVE pot from heat and stir in Gouda cheese, stirring until well combined. Let stand 1 minute to thicken before serving.

SIDES

WHAT MAKES IT QUICK & EASY: By using my Helpful Tip, this recipe can be prepped and cooked in only 10 minutes.

Calories: 180 · Fat: 13g · Protein: 9.5g · Total Carbs: 8g – Fiber: 3g = **Net Carbs: 5g**

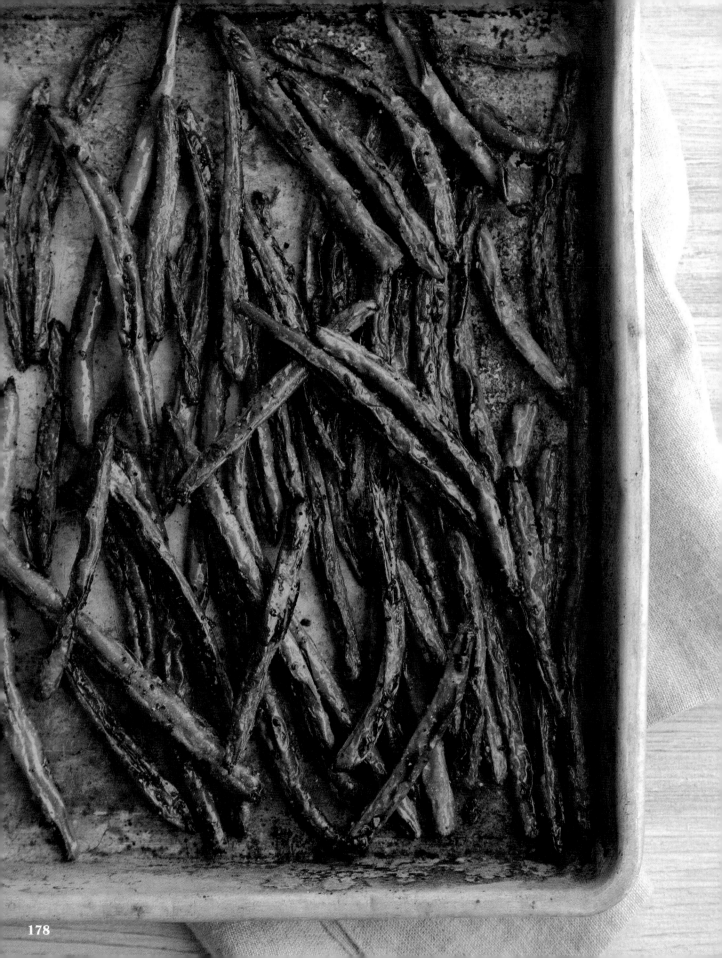

BROILED GREEN BEANS

CARAMELIZED GREEN BEANS WITH A NUTTY FLAVOR

Green beans naturally (and magically) take on an astonishing nuttiness when they caramelize in this recipe. Broiling under high heat allows the outside of the beans to brown, while still retaining a bit of crunch.

SHOPPING LIST

1 pound green beans, ends snapped

1 tablespoon olive oil

¼ teaspoon garlic powder

¼ teaspoon onion powder

¼ teaspoon salt

¼ teaspoon black pepper

HELPFUL TIPS

You can usually purchase steam bags of green beans in the produce section that have already had their ends snapped and removed.

1 SET broiler to high-heat.

2 IN a large mixing bowl, toss green beans with all remaining ingredients, evenly coating with the olive oil and spices.

3 ARRANGE the coated green beans on a sheet pan in a single layer.

4 BROIL for 10 minutes, flipping halfway through. Green beans are done when they are well browned. Serve immediately.

WHAT MAKES IT QUICK & EASY: With only 10 minutes under the broiler, these take only a few minutes longer than microwave-steaming green beans, but with FAR more flavor.

Calories: 65 • Fat: 3.5g • Protein: 2g • Total Carbs: 8g – Fiber: 4g = **Net Carbs: 4g**

SIDES

FRESH RATATOUILLE SAUTÉ

TRADITIONAL FLAVORS, WITHOUT THE WAIT

It can take quite a while to make the perfect stew, oftentimes requiring a laundry list of ingredients and steps, which is why I've come up with a way to prepare this iconic dish with as little effort as possible, while still keeping all the familiar flavors intact.

SHOPPING LIST

2 tablespoons olive oil

1 small eggplant, cut into 1-inch cubes

2 medium zucchini, chopped

1 large tomato, chopped

½ red onion, chopped large

½ yellow bell pepper, chopped

3 tablespoons chopped fresh basil

1 tablespoon minced garlic

1 teaspoon dried thyme

1 bay leaf

½ teaspoon salt

½ teaspoon black pepper

1 HEAT olive oil in a large skillet or Dutch oven over medium-high heat, until nearly smoking hot.

2 ADD all remaining ingredients to the skillet and stir to combine.

3 SAUTÉ, stirring occasionally for 5 minutes.

4 REDUCE heat to medium-low, cover, and cook for 15 minutes, uncovering only to stir occasionally, until eggplant is soft. Season with any additional salt and pepper to taste and remove bay leaf before serving.

HELPFUL TIPS

If the ratatouille begins to caramelize and stick to the bottom of the pot, simply add a splash of water. Personally, I love caramelization on vegetables.

WHAT MAKES IT QUICK & EASY: Traditional ratatouille is typically stewed for well over an hour, which this recipe cuts down to only 20 minutes.

Calories: 120 • Fat: 7.5g • Protein: 3g • Total Carbs: 12.5g – Fiber: 5.5g = **Net Carbs: 7g**

SIDES

SAVORY BALSAMIC MUSHROOMS
THE PERFECT TOPPER FOR STEAK AND PORK

Never again will you break out that bottle of sugar-filled steak sauce from the fridge, not after you've topped a prime cut with a few of these mushrooms. Balsamic has a way of bringing the best out of any red meat.

SHOPPING LIST

2 teaspoons olive oil

8 ounces sliced baby bella mushrooms

1 teaspoon minced garlic

½ teaspoon dried rosemary

¼ teaspoon black pepper

2 tablespoons balsamic vinegar

1 teaspoon beef base (see tip)

2 tablespoons unsalted butter

HELPFUL TIPS

Beef base can be purchased in small jars near the stocks and broths in the grocery store. Because it is concentrated, you can add far more beef flavor than simply adding stock.

1 HEAT oil in a large skillet over medium-high heat, until nearly smoking hot.

2 PLACE mushrooms, garlic, and rosemary in the hot skillet and sauté 5 minutes, or until mushrooms begin to brown.

3 REDUCE heat to medium-low, and add balsamic vinegar and beef base to the skillet. Stir to combine with mushrooms, and let simmer 1 minute.

4 REMOVE skillet from heat, and stir butter into the balsamic vinegar to thicken. Let rest 2 minutes before serving.

WHAT MAKES IT QUICK & EASY: This is a quick topping you can whip up to turn any cut of meat into a flavorful entrée in minutes.

Calories: 90 • Fat: 8g • Protein: 1.5g • Total Carbs: 3g – Fiber: 1g = **Net Carbs: 2g**

SIDES

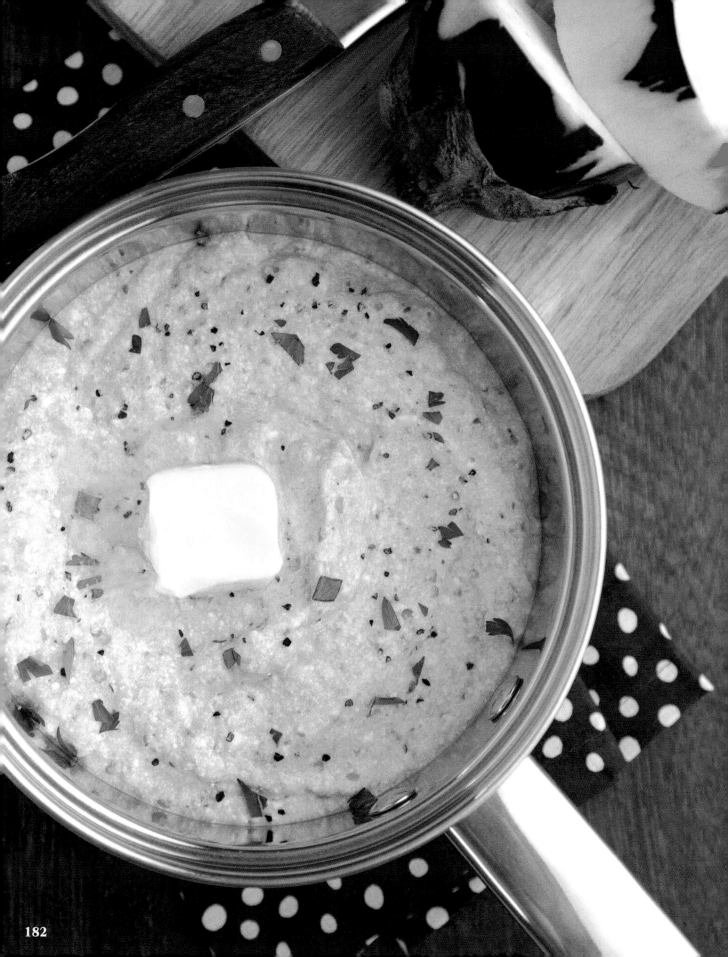

CREAMY EGGPLANT "POLENTA"

EGGPLANT PURÉE WITH RICOTTA CHEESE

While it might be one of the oddest fruits on the planet, and may sometimes stump some home cooks as to what to do with it, eggplant is surprisingly versatile. In fact, I'd bet my sharpest knife you never expected it could take the place of cornmeal, but it certainly can, and here's the proof.

SHOPPING LIST

1 medium eggplant

1 tablespoon unsalted butter

1 tablespoon olive oil

1 cup ricotta cheese

2 tablespoons grated Parmesan cheese

½ teaspoon garlic powder

½ teaspoon salt

¼ teaspoon black pepper

HELPFUL TIPS

Be sure to peel the eggplant before slicing off the ends, this way you don't have to get every bit of peel near the top and bottom, as they will be removed anyway.

1 PEEL eggplant, remove ends, and chop into 1-inch pieces.

2 PLACE butter, olive oil, and chopped eggplant in a large nonstick skillet over medium heat. Cover and let cook, stirring occasionally, for 12 minutes, or until tender.

3 TRANSFER cooked eggplant to a food processor or blender, and process until smooth.

4 RETURN the puréed eggplant to the skillet, and place over medium-low heat.

5 ADD all remaining ingredients, stirring to combine.

6 LET cook, stirring occasionally, for 3 minutes, just until warmed throughout. Serve immediately.

SIDES

WHAT MAKES IT QUICK & EASY: This cooks in half the time of traditional corn polenta.

Calories: 180 • Fat: 12.5g • Protein: 9.5g • Total Carbs: 9g – Fiber: 3.5g = **Net Carbs: 5.5g**

SIMPLY SAUTÉED BROCCOLI
WITH BUTTER AND SHALLOTS

You can't master the kitchen without first mastering how to make what is arguably the most popular vegetable—broccoli! This simple sauté may be basic, but it's far more flavorful than simply steaming.

SHOPPING LIST

2 tablespoons unsalted butter

16 ounces broccoli florets

1 large shallot, diced

¼ cup chicken stock

¼ teaspoon salt

¼ teaspoon pepper

1 HEAT butter in a large skillet over medium heat, until sizzling.

2 PLACE broccoli florets and diced shallot in the hot skillet and sauté 4 minutes.

3 ADD all remaining ingredients to the skillet and continue sautéing for 6 additional minutes, or until broccoli is crisp-tender. Serve immediately.

HELPFUL TIPS

You can use 3 tablespoons of diced red onion and 1½ teaspoons of minced garlic in place of the shallot in this recipe.

SIDES

WHAT MAKES IT QUICK & EASY: There's nothing simpler than a simple sauté!

Calories: 95 • Fat: 6g • Protein: 3.5g • Total Carbs: 9g − Fiber: 3g = **Net Carbs: 6g**

ROASTED TURNIPS

A LOW-CARB ROOT VEGETABLE GETS ITS DAY

Though most root vegetables are typically very high in carbs, turnips are actually lower in carbs than many green vegetables! Amazingly, this is the first time I've given them a starring role in a recipe, but it's a real winner. Once roasted, turnips make an amazing alternative to roasted potatoes to serve alongside beef, pork, or chicken.

SHOPPING LIST

Nonstick cooking spray

3 turnips, ends trimmed, peeled, and chopped

1 tablespoon olive oil

1 tablespoon balsamic vinegar

½ teaspoon dried rosemary

¼ teaspoon salt

¼ teaspoon black pepper

HELPFUL TIPS

In winter, these are very good when made by substituting 2 teaspoons of cider vinegar for the balsamic vinegar and ½ teaspoon of ground cinnamon in place of the rosemary.

1 PREHEAT oven to 450°F. Spray a sheet pan with nonstick cooking spray.

2 IN a large mixing bowl, toss turnips with all remaining ingredients to evenly coat.

3 ARRANGE the coated turnips on the prepared sheet pan in a single layer.

4 BAKE for 35 minutes, flipping halfway through. Turnips are done when golden brown and fork-tender. Season with additional salt to taste before serving.

SIDES

WHAT MAKES IT QUICK & EASY: The bake time on this recipe is longer than most sides, but this is a special occasion recipe we love around the holidays, so we decided to include it.

Calories: 55 • Fat: 3.5g • Protein: 1g • Total Carbs: 6g − Fiber: 1.5g = **Net Carbs: 4.5g**

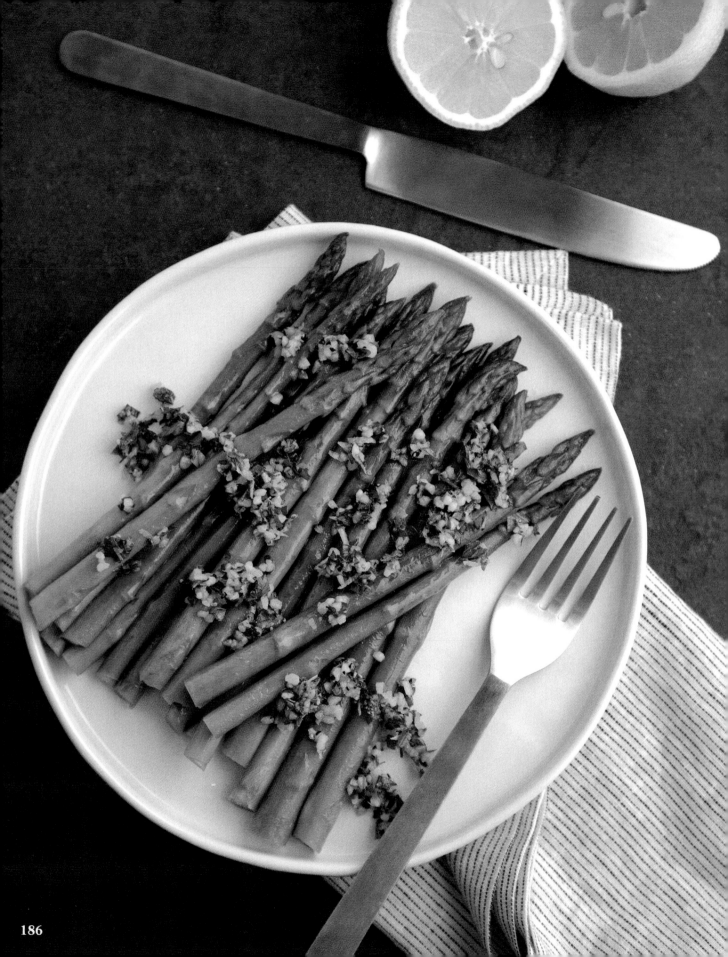

ASPARAGUS WITH GREMOLATA

ASPARAGUS WITH LEMON ZEST, PARSLEY, AND GARLIC

A little goes a long way with this easy-to-prepare gremolata. The bright and herby flavors lend a refreshing approach to asparagus, and pairs well with a great number of main courses.

SHOPPING LIST

1 pound asparagus, 2-inches trimmed from stalks

1 tablespoon olive oil

⅓ cup water

¼ teaspoon salt

GREMOLATA:

⅓ cup fresh parsley, finely chopped

Zest of 1 lemon

1½ teaspoons minced garlic

½ teaspoon olive oil

Salt and black pepper

1 PLACE asparagus, olive oil, water, and salt in a skillet over medium-high heat.

2 COVER and bring up to a simmer. Reduce heat to medium and let simmer for 6–8 minutes, just until asparagus is crisp-tender.

3 MEANWHILE, in a small mixing bowl, combine all Gremolata ingredients.

4 USE tongs to remove asparagus from any liquid in the skillet, transferring to a serving dish. Sprinkle the Gremolata over asparagus before serving.

HELPFUL TIPS

I prefer to make this with jarred minced garlic, as it is not as strong as fresh garlic, and the Gremolata does not get cooked to tone the garlic down.

WHAT MAKES IT QUICK & EASY: Gremolata is a quick condiment that you can prepare from pantry ingredients any time.

Calories: 60 · Fat: 4g · Protein: 2.5g · Total Carbs: 5.5g – Fiber: 2.5g = **Net Carbs: 3g**

SIDES

"PASTA" ALFREDO

MADE WITH ANY OF MY PASTA ALTERNATIVES

I'm not sure who Alfredo is, but I do know that his pasta is a true comfort food that the whole family loves. This recipe for low-carb Alfredo Sauce allows you to choose your Pasta Alternative of choice to make it your own. Nutritional information at bottom of page is for the sauce without any Pasta Alternative added.

SHOPPING LIST

2 tablespoons unsalted butter, divided

½ teaspoon minced garlic

1 cup heavy cream

½ teaspoon cracked black pepper

Pinch ground nutmeg

¾ cup grated Parmesan cheese

Salt

1 batch any Pasta Alternative, recipes page: 170–171

Chopped parsley, for garnish, if desired

HELPFUL TIPS

Top this with a grilled or pan-seared chicken breast for a complete meal.

1 HEAT 1 tablespoon of the butter and the minced garlic in a sauce pot over medium-high heat, until sizzling.

2 REDUCE heat to medium and stir in heavy cream, pepper, and nutmeg.

3 BRING the heavy cream to a simmer. Stirring frequently, let simmer for 5 minutes.

4 REMOVE pot from heat and whisk in Parmesan cheese and remaining 1 tablespoon of butter. Season with salt to taste.

5 LET stand 1 minute to thicken before tossing with your Pasta Alternative of choice. Garnish with chopped parsley, if desired.

WHAT MAKES IT QUICK & EASY: This family-favorite sauce is made entirely out of low-carb pantry staples!

Calories: 245 • Fat: 23.5g • Protein: 9.5g • Total Carbs: 1g – Fiber: 0g = **Net Carbs: 1g**

SIDES

SUMMER SQUASH SCAMPI

BUTTERY YELLOW SQUASH WITH LEMON AND GARLIC

Scampi isn't just for shrimp! Butter, lemon, and garlic combine to perfectly complement tender yellow squash in this easy sauté that doesn't skimp on flavor.

SHOPPING LIST

3 tablespoons unsalted butter

4 large yellow squash, thinly sliced into discs

¼ cup diced red onion

Juice of ½ lemon

2 teaspoons minced garlic

¼ teaspoon garlic powder

¼ teaspoon salt

¼ teaspoon black pepper

1 tablespoon chopped parsley

1 HEAT butter in a large skillet over medium heat, until sizzling.

2 PLACE yellow squash and red onion in the hot skillet and sauté 3 minutes.

3 ADD all remaining ingredients, except parsley, to the skillet and continue sautéing for 4 additional minutes, or until yellow squash is crisp-tender.

4 TOP with chopped parsley before serving immediately.

HELPFUL TIPS

Generally, yellow squash and zucchini are interchangeable so feel free to use zucchini or a mix of yellow squash and zucchini in this recipe.

WHAT MAKES IT QUICK & EASY: This simple side is cooked in only 7 minutes.

Calories: 110 • Fat: 9g • Protein: 2g • Total Carbs: 7g – Fiber: 2g = **Net Carbs: 5g**

SIDES

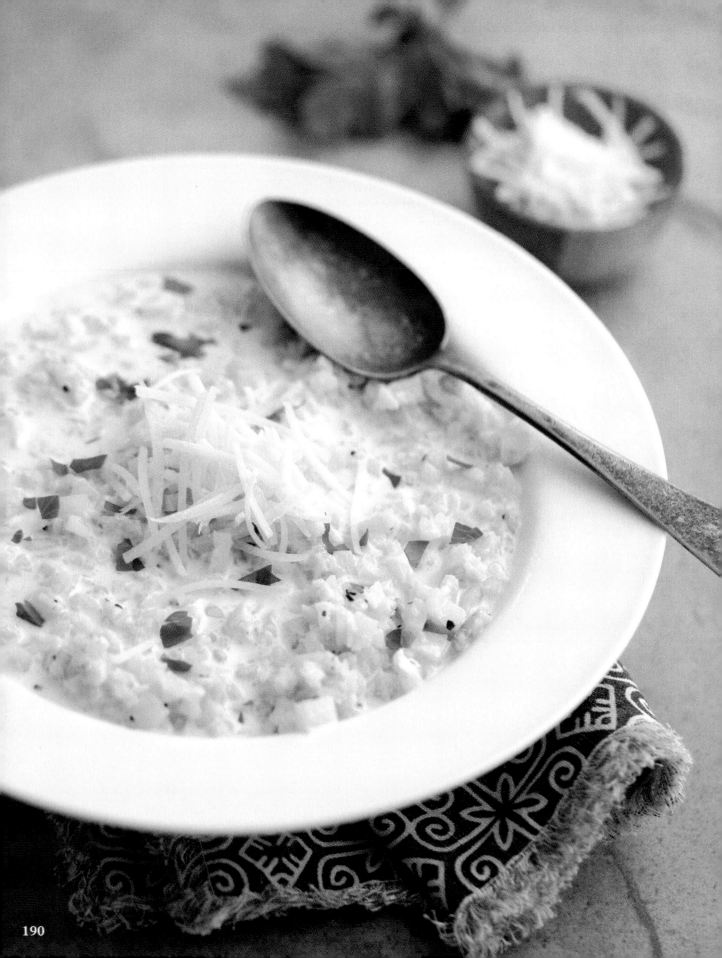

CAULIFLOWER RISOTTO

A CREAMY RE-INVENTION OF A CLASSIC RICE DISH

It seems to me that anywhere you go these days, every restaurant has its own unique take on risotto. As a chef, I've made many versions. Here, crumbled cauliflower replaces the traditional rice, cutting the carbs down to the minimum while still maintaining that rich and creamy consistency we have come to know and love.

SHOPPING LIST

1 tablespoon olive oil

1 medium head cauliflower, grated (see tip)

1 small shallot, finely diced

2 teaspoons minced garlic

½ cup chicken stock

¼ cup dry white wine (may use additional chicken stock)

¼ teaspoon salt

¼ teaspoon black pepper

⅓ cup heavy cream

⅓ cup grated Parmesan cheese

Chopped parsley, for garnish, if desired

1 HEAT olive oil in a nonstick skillet over medium-high heat, until nearly smoking hot.

2 ADD cauliflower, shallot, and minced garlic to the skillet and sauté 3 minutes.

3 ADD chicken stock, white wine, salt, and pepper to the skillet, and let simmer 3 minutes.

4 STIR in heavy cream, and simmer an additional 3 minutes.

5 REMOVE from heat, and stir in Parmesan cheese. Let rest 3 minutes, to thicken, before serving garnished with chopped parsley, if desired.

HELPFUL TIPS

To make cauliflower crumbles, you can grate cauliflower using the large holes of a cheese grater. That said, Green Giant now sell bags of cauliflower crumbles! One bag equals about 1 head of cauliflower, the perfect amount for this recipe.

SIDES

WHAT MAKES IT QUICK & EASY: This cooks in about half the time of traditional risotto, and without the need to constantly stir.

Calories: 155 • Fat: 10.5g • Protein: 6.5g • Total Carbs: 8.5g – Fiber: 3g = **Net Carbs: 5.5g**

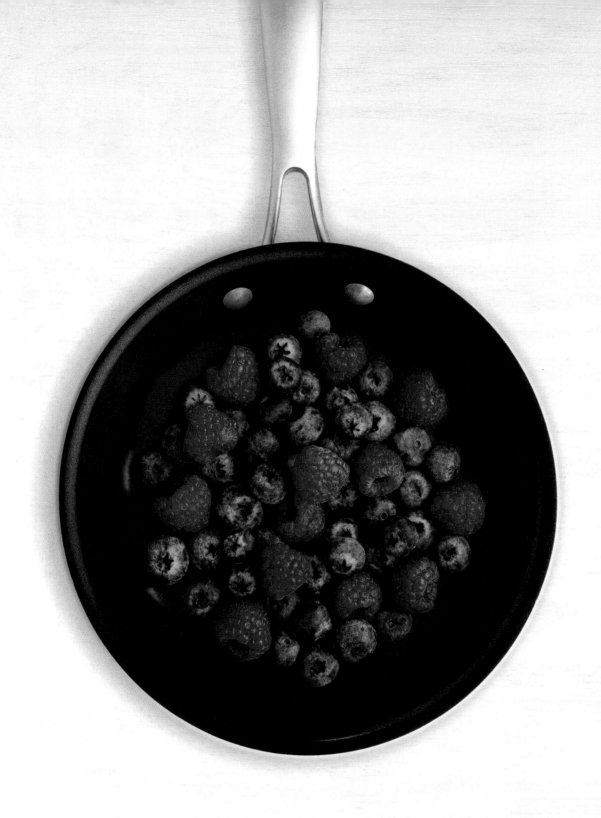

DESSERTS

~~~~~~~~~~~~~~

DESSERTS

QUICK & EASY DESSERT STAPLES

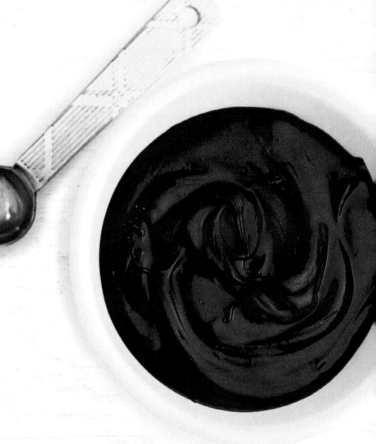

CHOCOLATE GANACHE

8 SERVINGS

1 tablespoon unsalted butter

½ cup sugar substitute

2 teaspoons half-and-half

1 ounce unsweetened baking chocolate, chopped

1 teaspoon vanilla extract

1 FILL a small pot with 2 inches of water and bring to a simmer over medium-high heat.

2 PLACE a stainless steel or tempered glass bowl over the pot to create a double-boiler.

3 ADD the butter, sugar substitute, and half-and-half to the bowl of the double-boiler and mix with a silicone spatula, until combined.

4 ADD the chocolate and stir constantly, just until the chocolate has melted and all is combined.

5 REMOVE from heat and stir in vanilla extract. Use ganache immediately, while still warm.

Calories: 40 • Fat: 3.5g • Protein: 0.5g
Total Carbs: 2.5g – Fiber: 0.5g = **Net Carbs: 2g**

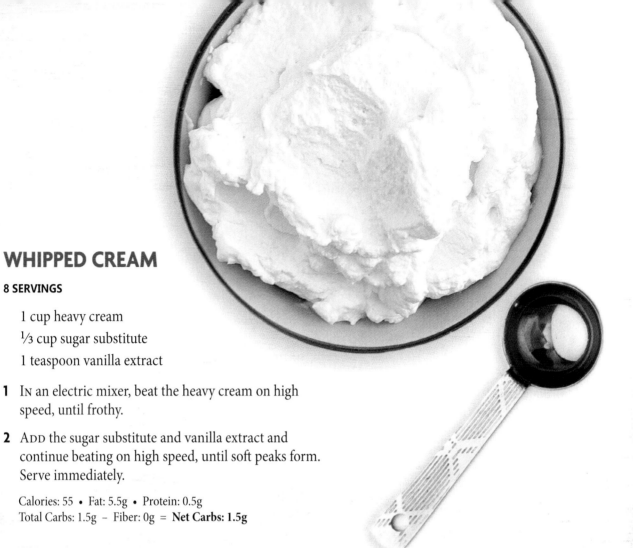

WHIPPED CREAM

8 SERVINGS

1 cup heavy cream

⅓ cup sugar substitute

1 teaspoon vanilla extract

1 IN an electric mixer, beat the heavy cream on high speed, until frothy.

2 ADD the sugar substitute and vanilla extract and continue beating on high speed, until soft peaks form. Serve immediately.

Calories: 55 • Fat: 5.5g • Protein: 0.5g
Total Carbs: 1.5g – Fiber: 0g = **Net Carbs: 1.5g**

BUTTERCREAM CHEESE FROSTING

8 SERVINGS

8 ounces cream cheese, softened

½ cup sugar substitute

4 tablespoons unsalted butter, softened

1 teaspoon vanilla extract

1 IN an electric mixer, beat all ingredients on high speed until light and fluffy.

2 SPREAD on cooled baked goods. Store refrigerated.

Calories: 155 • Fat: 15.5g • Protein: 2g
Total Carbs: 2g – Fiber: 0g = **Net Carbs: 2g**

DESSERTS

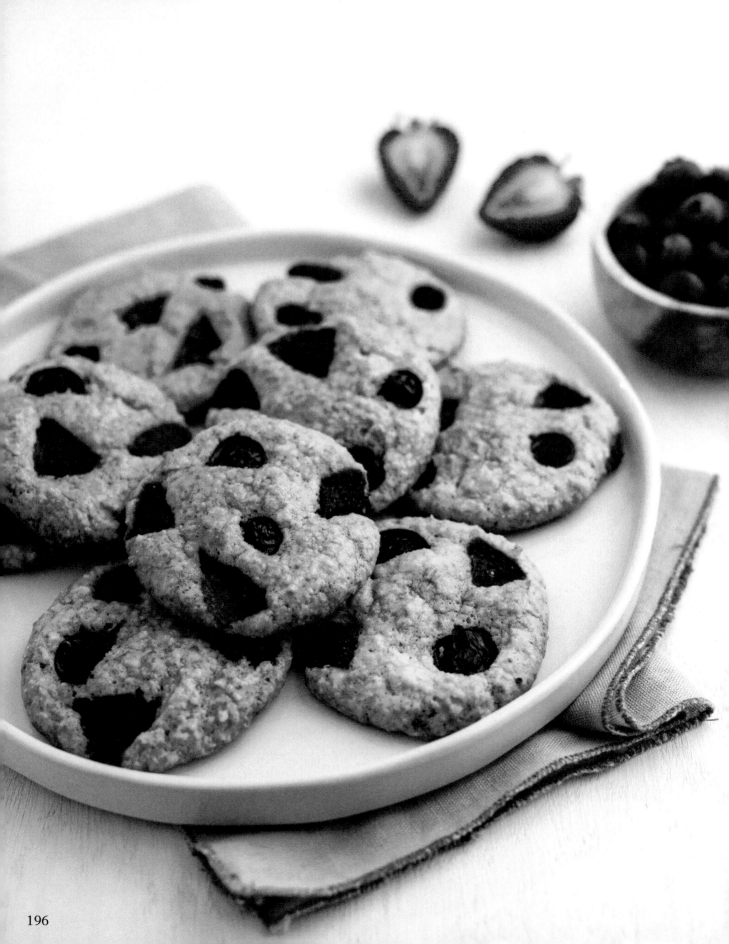

BERRY & CREAM CHEESE COOKIES
RED, WHITE, AND BLUE FOR THE SWEET TOOTH IN YOU

These cookies have the flavor of a cream cheese Danish with a beautiful and patriotic presentation thanks to fresh strawberries and blueberries. They make the perfect dessert for an Independence Day picnic, or any picnic, or any weeknight—or breakfast the next morning.

SHOPPING LIST

2 ounces cream cheese, softened

2 tablespoons unsalted butter, softened

1 cup sugar substitute

1 large egg

1 teaspoon vanilla extract

1 cup blanched almond flour

½ teaspoon baking soda

Pinch salt

¼ cup chopped fresh strawberries

¼ cup fresh blueberries (see tip)

HELPFUL TIPS

Small blueberries work best in this recipe, so that they do not stick too far out of the cookies. Larger blueberries can be cut in half to make for the best looking cookie.

1 PREHEAT oven to 375°F. Line a sheet pan with parchment paper.

2 ADD the cream cheese, butter, sugar substitute, egg, and vanilla extract to an electric mixer. Set to high and mix until creamy and fluffy.

3 ADD the almond flour, baking soda, and salt to the mixer and mix on medium until well blended.

4 USING a tablespoon or 1-ounce ice cream scoop, drop 16 evenly-spaced cookies onto the prepared sheet pan. Lightly tap the pan on the counter to flatten cookies.

5 LIGHLY press a few of each berry into each cookie.

6 BAKE for 13–14 minutes, just until the bottom of the cookies are golden brown. Let cool for 10 minutes before serving.

WHAT MAKES IT QUICK & EASY: While it may look like a lot of ingredients, nearly all of them are staples of any low-carb pantry.

Calories: 155 · Fat: 13g · Protein: 4.5g · Total Carbs: 7g – Fiber: 1.5g = **Net Carbs: 5.5g**

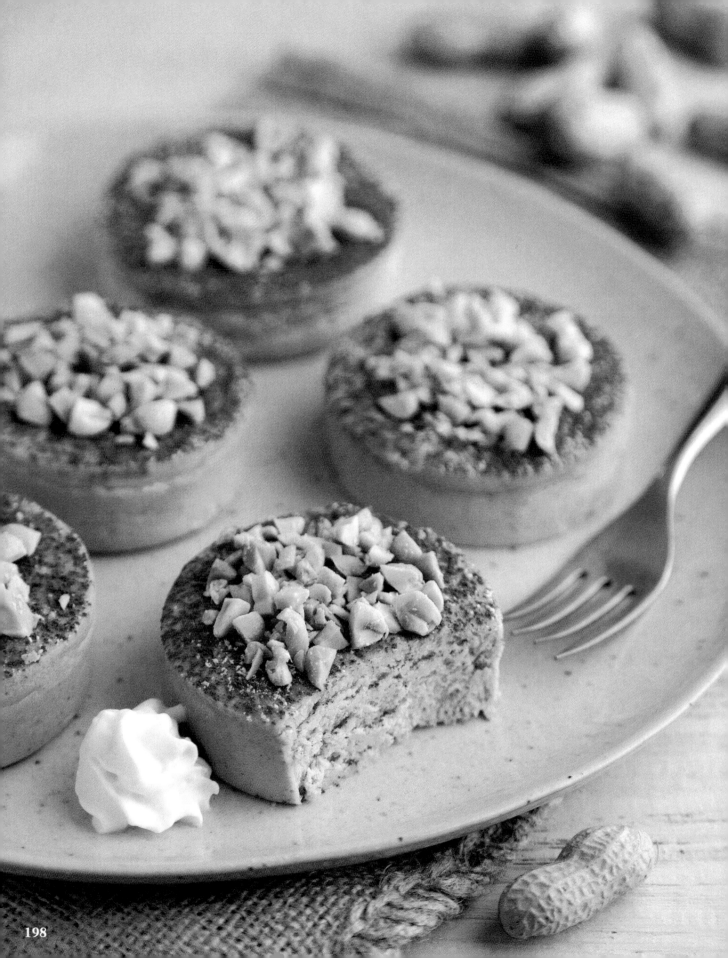

PEANUT BUTTER CHEESECAKE MINIS
OUR QUICKEST, EASIEST CHEESECAKE RECIPE EVER

All natural peanut butter is mixed right into the batter of these crustless mini cheesecakes. By baking them in individual serving cups, you can really cut down on the typically long cook times of traditional cheesecakes.

SHOPPING LIST

Nonstick cooking spray

12 ounces cream cheese, softened

½ cup sugar substitute

⅓ cup natural smooth peanut butter

2 large eggs

2 tablespoons half-and-half

2 teaspoons vanilla extract

HELPFUL TIPS

We like to garnish these with a sprinkling of unsweetened cocoa powder, chopped peanuts, and a dollop of sugar-free whipped cream.

1 PLACE oven rack in the center position and preheat to 350°F. Spray 6 (6-ounce) ramekins or oven-safe custard cups with nonstick cooking spray.

2 MAKE a water bath by pouring ¾ inch of hot water into a shallow roasting pan. Place the water bath onto the center oven rack to preheat.

3 PLACE all ingredients in an electric mixer, and mix on medium speed, just until combined.

4 SPREAD an equal amount of filling into each of the 6 ramekins.

5 PLACE the ramekins in the preheated water bath, and bake for 26–28 minutes, just until the tops of the cheesecakes start to crack.

6 COOL on a wire rack for 30 minutes, then refrigerate at least 1½ hours before serving.

DESSERTS

WHAT MAKES IT QUICK & EASY: Cheesecake baked in under 30 minutes?! I'd think it was crazy if I didn't bake it myself!

Calories: 330 • Fat: 29g • Protein: 9.5g • Total Carbs: 6.5g − Fiber: 1g = **Net Carbs: 5.5g**

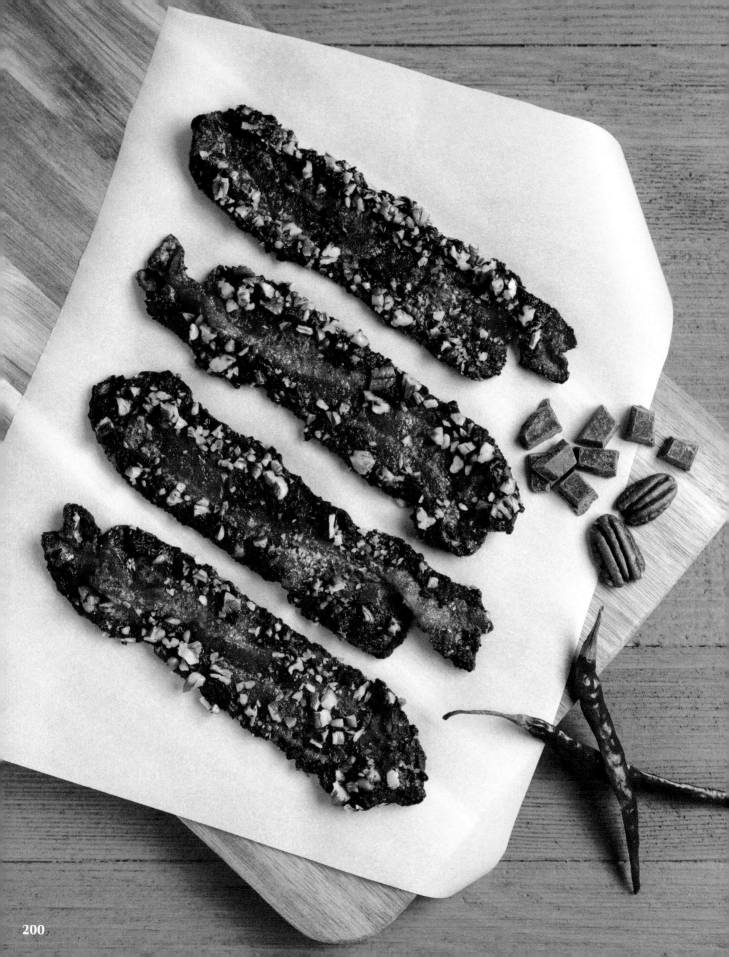

CHOCOLATE MAPLE BACON

ALSO KNOWN AS "PIG CANDY"

No savory ingredient goes better with dessert than bacon! In this recipe, not only do I candy the bacon with maple, but then I dip it in chocolate and pecans to really take the indulgence to another level. A hint of ground cayenne pepper adds a little spice (although you can choose to leave this out), as chili peppers also go great with chocolate.

SHOPPING LIST

8 slices thick-cut bacon

¼ cup sugar substitute

2 tablespoons unsalted butter, melted

1 teaspoon maple extract

¼ teaspoon ground cayenne pepper, optional

1 batch Chocolate Ganache, recipe page: 194

¼ cup finely chopped pecans

HELPFUL TIPS

You can also make this as simply Maple Candied Bacon and omit coating the slices in Chocolate Ganache and pecans. Simply stop after step 4. The candied bacon is really good all on its own.

1 PREHEAT oven to 375°F. Line a sheet pan with parchment paper.

2 LAY the bacon out on the lined sheet pan.

3 IN a small bowl, mix the sugar substitute, melted butter, maple extract, and cayenne pepper. Spoon mixture evenly over the top of each bacon slice.

4 BAKE for 20–30 minutes, until bacon is crispy (cooking time will vary dramatically based on thickness of bacon).

5 TRANSFER cooked bacon to paper towels and refrigerate as you prepare the Ganache.

6 PREPARE the Chocolate Ganache according to the directions.

7 DIP the outer edges of the cooked bacon into the warm Ganache, and then immediately press into the chopped pecans. Transfer to a parchment lined plate. Repeat until all 8 slices are coated.

8 CHILL 30 minutes to set the chocolate before serving.

DESSERTS

WHAT MAKES IT QUICK & EASY: See tip for an even easier sweet and savory treat.

Calories: 185 • Fat: 16g • Protein: 5g • Total Carbs: 3.5g − Fiber: 0.5g = **Net Carbs: 3g**

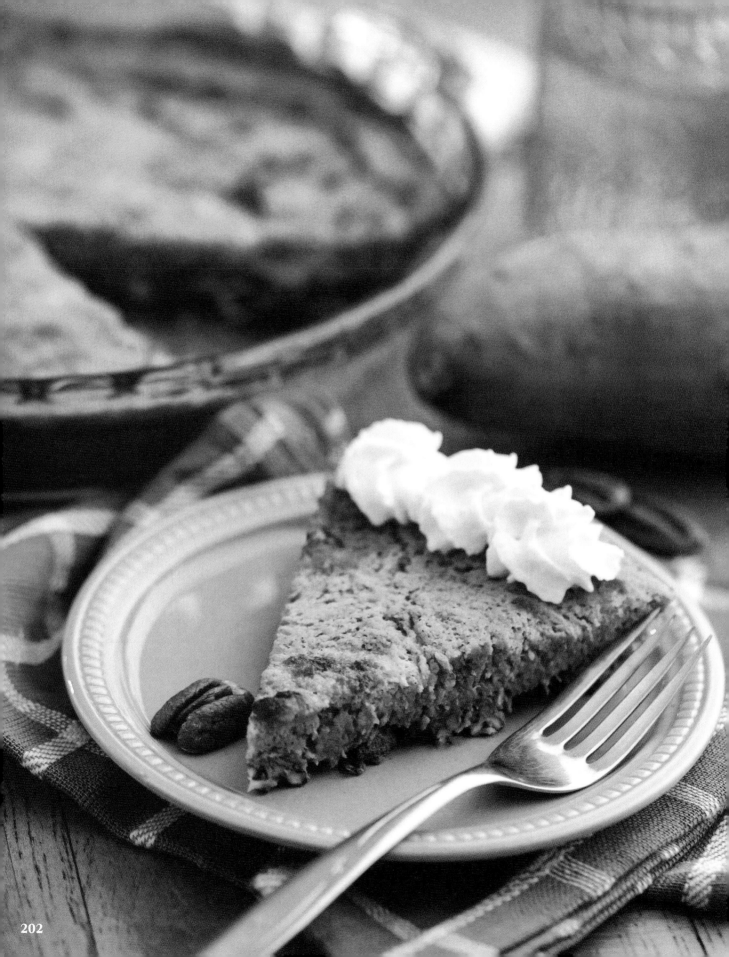

SWEET POTATO PIE
STRETCHED WITH MERINGUE TO LOWER THE CARBS

I've lowered the carbs of this Southern staple by folding meringue into the sweet potato filling. It not only helps hold the pie together, but bulks it up, allowing you to use less potato without losing flavor.

SHOPPING LIST

Nonstick cooking spray

½ cup chopped pecans

MERINGUE

2 large egg whites, room temperature

2 tablespoons sugar substitute

¼ teaspoon cream of tartar

FILLING

3 large sweet potatoes, baked and cooled (see tip)

2 large egg yolks

¼ cup sugar substitute

1 tablespoon half-and-half

1 teaspoon vanilla extract

½ teaspoon pumpkin pie spice

HELPFUL TIPS

To cook sweet potatoes, poke with a fork in several places to vent steam. Bake at 400°F for 45 minutes, or microwave for 8–10 minutes until soft.

1 PREHEAT oven to 350°F. Spray a 9-inch deep dish pie plate with nonstick cooking spray. Line the bottom of the plate with the chopped pecans.

2 ADD all Meringue ingredients to an electric mixer and beat on high for 3–4 minutes, until soft peaks form. Set aside.

3 START the Filling by slicing the baked sweet potatoes in half, and scooping the soft potato out of the skin with a spoon. Place in a clean mixing bowl, discarding skins.

4 ADD the remaining Filling ingredients to the sweet potato, and whisk until smooth.

5 USE a rubber spatula to fold the Meringue into the Filling, until all is combined. Spread into the prepared pie plate.

6 BAKE for 55 minutes, or until sticking a toothpick into the center comes out mostly clean. Cool on a wire rack for 30 minutes, then refrigerate for 3 hours before slicing to serve.

DESSERTS

WHAT MAKES IT QUICK & EASY: This is arguably one of the most complicated recipes in the book, but making the crust out of only pecans instead of dough does simplify things.

Calories: 115 • Fat: 7g • Protein: 3.5g • Total Carbs: 11.5g – Fiber: 2.5g = **Net Carbs: 9g**

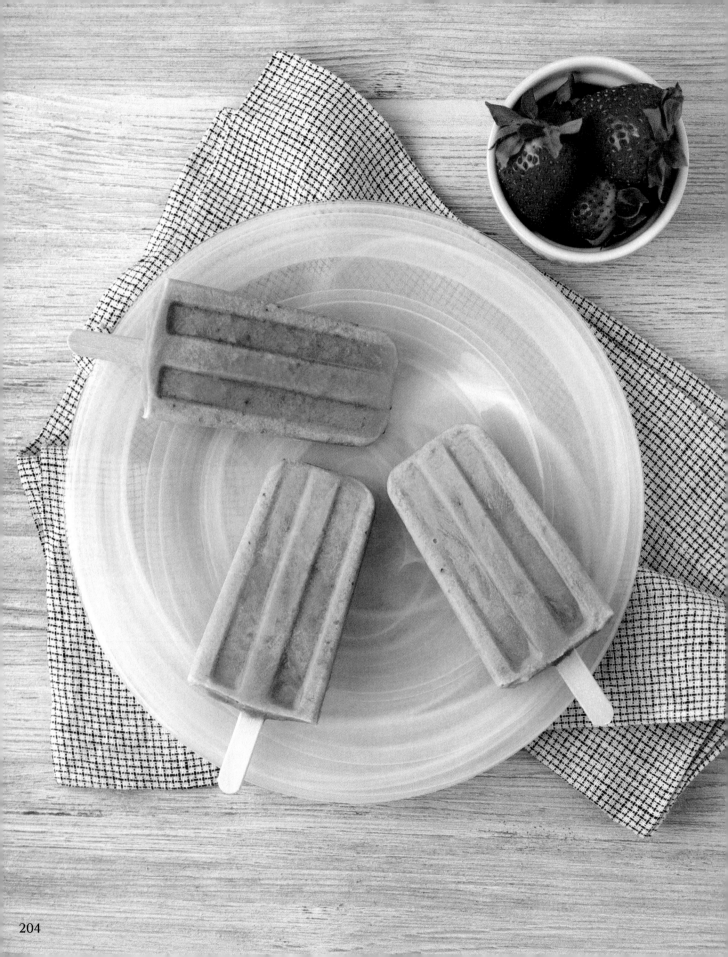

STRAWBERRY & CREAM ICE POPS
MADE FROM REAL STRAWBERRIES

These popsicles are made from a whole pint of fresh strawberries to pack the strawberry flavor, without the added sugar of traditional frozen fruit bars. A little heavy cream makes the pops a little creamier than your standard popsicle, and a whole lot better tasting!

SHOPPING LIST

16 ounces fresh strawberries, hulled

¾ cup water

⅓ cup heavy cream

⅓ cup sugar substitute

½ teaspoon vanilla extract

8 wooden pop sticks

HELPFUL TIPS

To easily release pops from their mold, dip the bottom of the mold in warm tap water for just a few seconds.

1 SET out an ice pop mold that can make at least 8 (3-ounce) pops.

2 ADD all ingredients, except wooden sticks, to a blender and blend until smooth.

3 POUR the mixture evenly between the 8 pop molds, filling each about ⅞ of the way full.

4 INSERT a wooden stick into each pop. Freeze for at least 3 hours, or until frozen solid.

DESSERTS

WHAT MAKES IT QUICK & EASY: Only a few seconds of blending, and you have homemade pops made from real strawberries.

Calories: 40 • Fat: 2g • Protein: 0.5g • Total Carbs: 5.5g – Fiber: 1g = **Net Carbs: 4.5g**

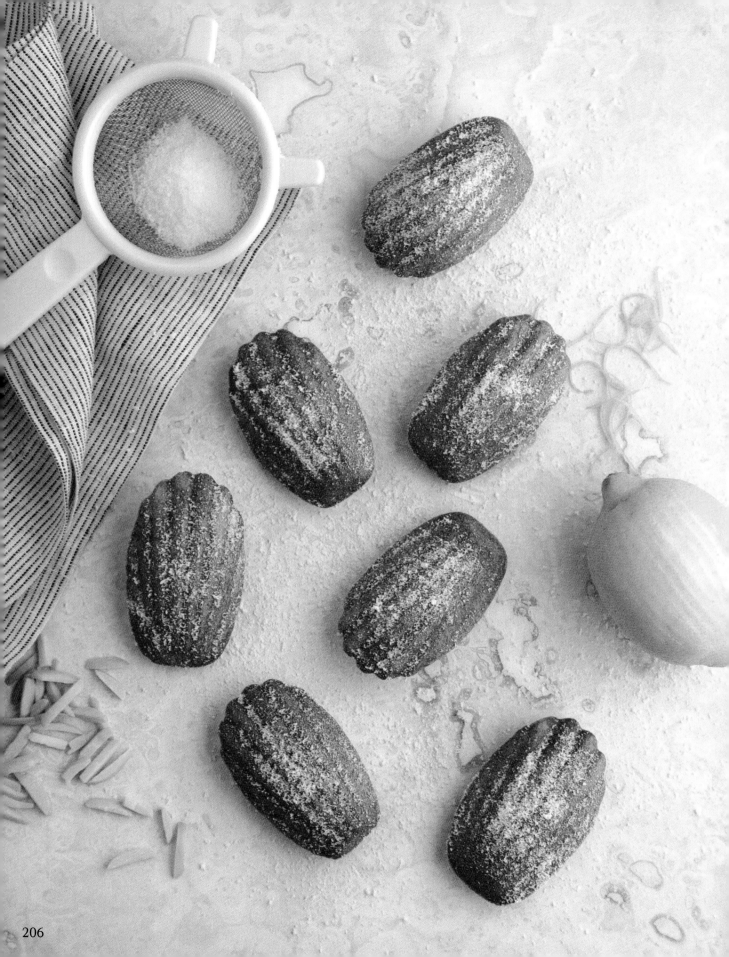

LEMON MADELEINES

LIGHT AND FLUFFY COOKIES WITH A CRISP CRUST

I love reinventing French desserts, as French pastry chefs often use almond flour as a secret ingredient to add more flavor to their desserts. It isn't a substitution over there, just another kitchen staple. Here I've used almond flour to reinvent French Madeleines; buttery cookies that are fluffy on the inside and crispy on the outside.

SHOPPING LIST

3 tablespoons unsalted butter, softened

½ cup sugar substitute

2 large eggs

1 large egg white

½ teaspoon vanilla extract

⅔ cup blanched almond flour

Zest of 1 lemon

½ teaspoon baking powder

HELPFUL TIPS

A regular madeleine pan has 12 molds that are about 3 inches each. Pans with 24 molds are typically mini madeleine pans, which you can also use, however you should check for doneness after only 7 minutes.

1 PREHEAT oven to 375°F. Set out a 12-mold standard-sized madeleine pan (see tip). If pan is not nonstick coated, spray with nonstick cooking spray.

2 ADD the butter, sugar substitute, egg, egg white, and vanilla extract to an electric mixer. Set to high, and mix until creamy and fluffy.

3 ADD the almond flour, lemon zest, and baking powder to the mixer and mix on medium until well blended.

4 USING a tablespoon, drop rounded spoonfuls of the batter evenly between the 12 madeleine molds, topping each off until all batter has been used. Lightly tap the pan on the counter to flatten out the batter and disperse within the molds.

5 BAKE for 10 minutes, just until the tops of the madeleines have puffed up and edges are golden brown. Let cool for at least 10 minutes before serving sprinkled with additional sugar substitute for garnish, if desired.

WHAT MAKES IT QUICK & EASY: By using the madeleine molds, you get perfectly even browning, a uniform shape, and an elegant presentation without any additional prep work.

Calories: 80 • Fat: 7g • Protein: 2.5g • Total Carbs: 2.5g – Fiber: 0.5g = **Net Carbs: 2g**

DESSERTS

MAPLE CAPPUCCINO PARFAITS
A WHIPPED DESSERT WITH TIRAMISU FLAVORS

This whipped up dessert reminds Rachel of "Coffee Milk," the state drink of Rhode Island, where she grew up. The combination of instant coffee and maple extract really tastes like coffee-flavored syrup that is used in that drink and many coffee desserts like tiramisu. While desserts like tiramisu should be made with real espresso, restaurants and bakeries often use the flavored coffee syrup, which is why you can't quite replicate the flavor at home.

SHOPPING LIST

1 tablespoon instant coffee granules

2 tablespoons hot water

¾ cup whole milk ricotta cheese

¾ cup heavy whipping cream

⅓ cup sugar substitute

1 teaspoon maple extract

1 teaspoon vanilla extract

1 DISSOLVE instant coffee in the 2 tablespoons of hot water.

2 ADD the dissolved coffee and all other ingredients to an electric mixer.

3 WHIP on high speed, just until soft peaks form. Be careful not to overwhip.

4 SPOON into 6 small parfait glasses and refrigerate for 1 hour before serving.

HELPFUL TIPS

My Lemon Madeleines, recipe page: 207, make an amazing cookie to serve stuck into each of these parfaits. You can even make the Madeleines without any lemon zest so that they are just buttery and sweet and don't overpower the flavors of the parfait.

DESSERTS

WHAT MAKES IT QUICK & EASY: This is a simple, but elegant dessert that can be prepared before dinner to serve 6 small, but rich portions.

Calories: 110 • Fat: 9g • Protein: 3g • Total Carbs: 4g − Fiber: 0g = **Net Carbs: 4g**

COCONUT MUG CAKE

A ONE-MINUTE MICROWAVE CAKE

This rapidly-rising coconut cake is packed full of heart-healthy omega-3s, thanks to ground flaxseeds. While the calories and fat may seem high, a good amount of that comes from the "good" fat of flax. Enjoy with or without frosting. Nutritional information is for the cake unfrosted.

SHOPPING LIST

¼ cup almond flour

1 large egg

1 tablespoon milled flaxseed (golden is best)

2 tablespoons sugar substitute

1 teaspoon unsalted butter, melted

½ teaspoon baking powder

½ teaspoon coconut extract

Buttercream Cheese Frosting, recipe page: 195, if desired

1 ADD all ingredients, except frosting, to a microwave-safe mug.

2 WHISK with a fork until well combined.

3 MICROWAVE for 1 minute on high, or until the batter rises in the mug and a toothpick inserted into the center comes out mostly clean.

4 TOP with a dollop of Buttercream Cheese Frosting, if desired. Or simply top with sugar-free whipped cream.

HELPFUL TIPS

If the cake is not entirely set, only cook for an additional 5–10 seconds at a time. These things cook fast! One minute always works perfect for us.

DESSERTS

WHAT MAKES IT QUICK & EASY: You can't make a cake any faster than this!

Calories: 360 • Fat: 29g • Protein: 15.5g • Total Carbs: 11g – Fiber: 7.5g = **Net Carbs: 3.5g**

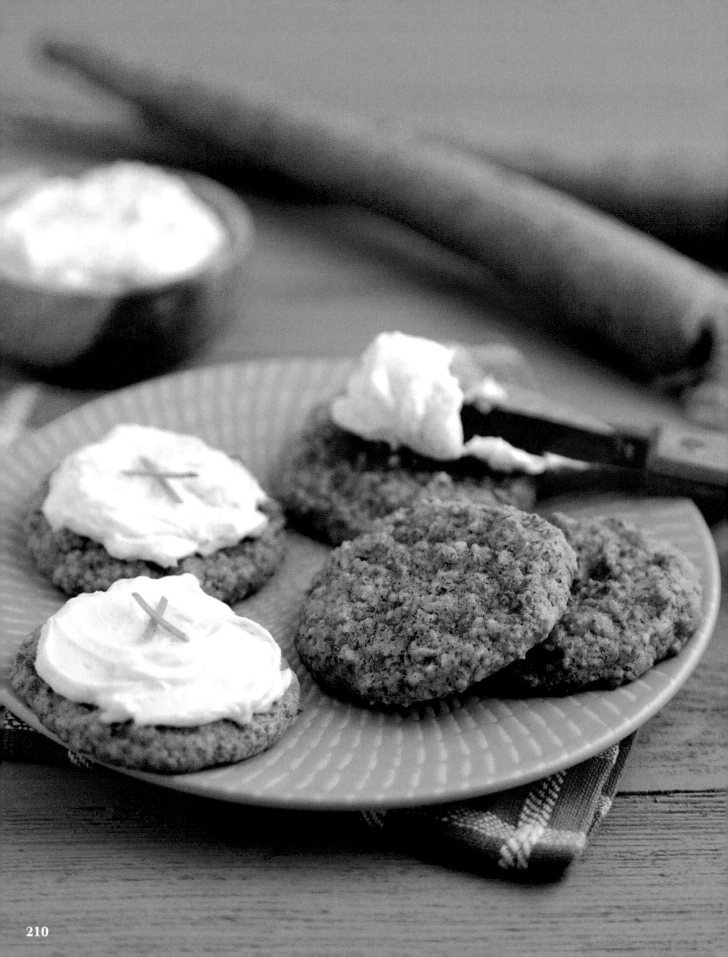

CARROT CAKE COOKIES

WITH OR WITHOUT FROSTING

With all the flavor of carrot cake, and fresh grated carrot throughout, these cookies hit the spot without the difficulty of baking and frosting an entire cake! As frosting is optional, nutritional information is for the cookies unfrosted.

SHOPPING LIST

2 ounces cream cheese, softened

2 tablespoons unsalted butter, softened

¾ cup sugar substitute

1 large egg

1 teaspoon vanilla extract

1 cup almond flour

½ teaspoon baking soda

½ teaspoon pumpkin pie spice

½ cup grated carrots (see tip)

½ cup finely chopped walnuts

½ batch Buttercream Cheese Frosting, recipe page: 195, if desired

HELPFUL TIPS

For those on a very restricted carb diet, the grated carrots (which contain natural sugars) can be omitted. Otherwise, use the smaller holes of a cheese grater to create the perfect consistency for this recipe.

1 PREHEAT oven to 375°F. Line two sheet pans with parchment paper.

2 ADD the cream cheese, butter, sugar substitute, egg, and vanilla extract to an electric mixer. Set to high and mix until creamy and fluffy.

3 ADD the almond flour, baking soda, and pumpkin pie spice to the mixer, and mix on medium, until blended into a dough.

4 FOLD the carrots and chopped walnuts into the dough.

5 USING a tablespoon or 1-ounce ice cream scoop, drop 20 evenly-spaced cookies onto the prepared sheet pans. Lightly press down on each cookie to flatten.

6 BAKE for 13–15 minutes, just until the bottom of the cookies are golden brown. Let cool for 10 minutes before serving, topped with Buttercream Cheese Frosting, if desired.

WHAT MAKES IT QUICK & EASY: While this may look like a lot of ingredients, nearly all of them are staples of any low-carb pantry.

DESSERTS

Calories: 160 · Fat: 14g · Protein: 5g · Total Carbs: 5.5g – Fiber: 2g = **Net Carbs: 3.5g**

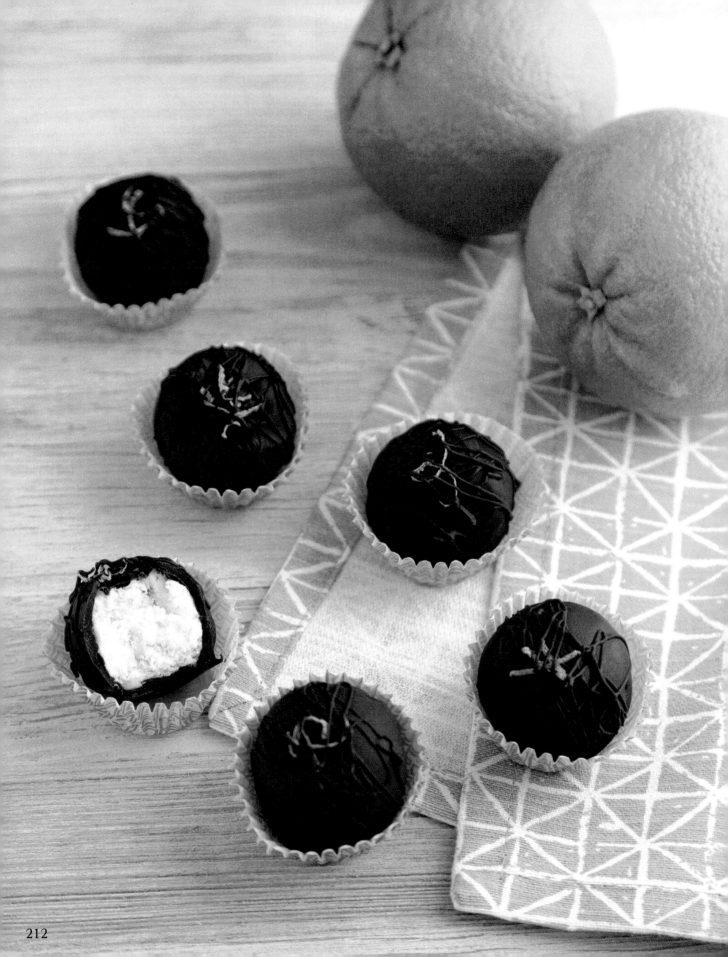

CREAMSICLE TRUFFLES

DARK CHOCOLATE TRUFFLES WITH ORANGE & CREAM FILLING

The filling of these chocolate treats taste just like an old favorite of mine—orange creamsicles. Unlike creamsicles, I've managed to achieve that zippy flavor using real orange zest.

SHOPPING LIST

6 ounces cream cheese, softened

3 tablespoons sugar substitute

2 teaspoons orange zest

½ teaspoon vanilla extract

1 batch Chocolate Ganache, recipe page: 194

HELPFUL TIPS

For a better presentation, sprinkle additional orange zest over the Chocolate Ganache directly after dipping.

1 LINE a small sheet pan or any freezer-safe dish with parchment paper.

2 IN a mixing bowl, use a fork to whisk together cream cheese, sugar substitute, orange zest, and vanilla extract.

3 FORM the mixture into 16 marble-sized balls. Place on the prepared sheet pan. Freeze for at least 30 minutes.

4 PREPARE the Chocolate Ganache according to the directions.

5 USING a fork, dip the frozen cream cheese balls, one at a time, into the warm ganache, spinning to coat. Work quickly before the chocolate cools. Place each coated truffle back onto the parchment-lined dish.

6 FREEZE an additional 30 minutes, until the chocolate has hardened. Serve chilled or frozen, as these tend to melt quickly.

DESSERTS

WHAT MAKES IT QUICK & EASY: Truffles like these are one of my go-to desserts, because I always have nearly all of the ingredients on hand.

Calories: 120 • Fat: 11g • Protein: 2g • Total Carbs: 4g – Fiber: 1g = **Net Carbs: 3.5g**

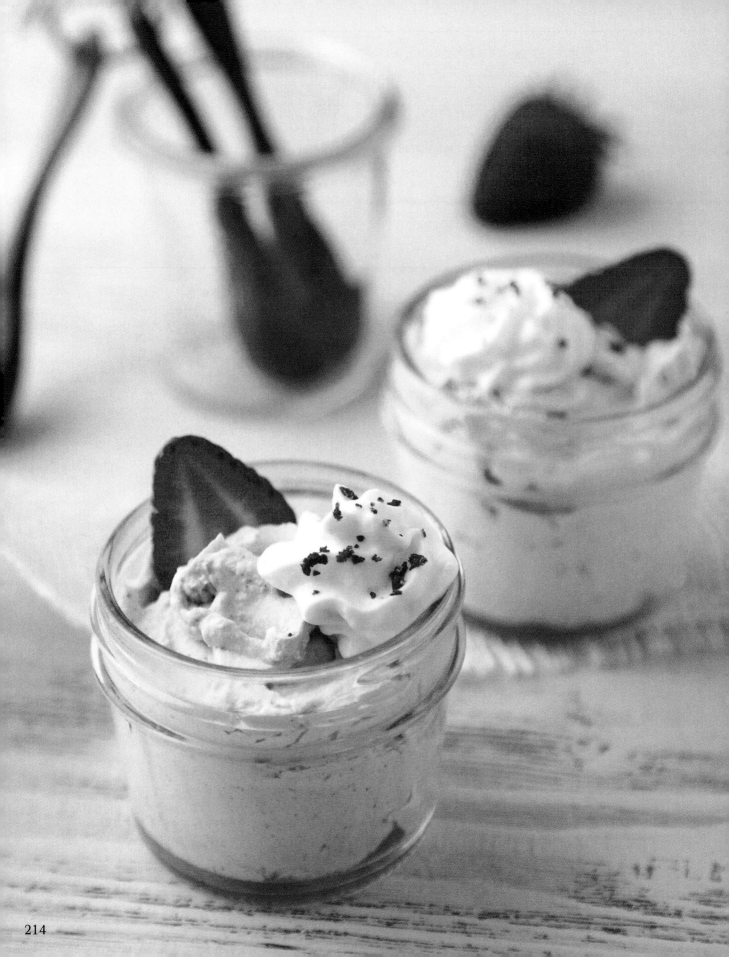

STRAWBERRY MOUSSE
A SIMPLE TRICK FOR FULL STRAWBERRY FLAVOR

This simple Strawberry Mousse packs an intense strawberry-punch, thanks to the concentrated flavor of freeze-dried strawberries that you food-process into a powder for easy mixing. You can usually find freeze-dried strawberries without any added sugar near the raisins and dried fruit in the grocery store, although they may also be located near the fancier dried fruit in the produce section.

SHOPPING LIST

½ cup freeze-dried strawberries
(see description above)

¾ cup heavy cream

⅓ cup sugar substitute

HELPFUL TIPS

For a nice presentation, save a pinch of the freeze-dried strawberry powder after food processing and sprinkle over the top of the mousse before serving.

1 PLACE freeze-dried strawberries in a food processor and process until they are a fine powder.

2 ADD heavy cream to the food processor and process only a few seconds, just to mix the cream with the strawberry powder.

3 TRANSFER to an electric mixer and mix on high speed, until frothy.

4 ADD the sugar substitute to the mixer and continue beating on high speed, until more than double in volume and hard peaks form. Serve immediately. Garnish with sugar-free whipped cream and fresh strawberries, if desired.

WHAT MAKES IT QUICK & EASY: Only three ingredients, and only a single non-pantry ingredient make this a dessert you can whip up any time.

Calories: 130 • Fat: 11.5g • Protein: 1g • Total Carbs: 6g − Fiber: 0.5g = **Net Carbs: 5.5g**

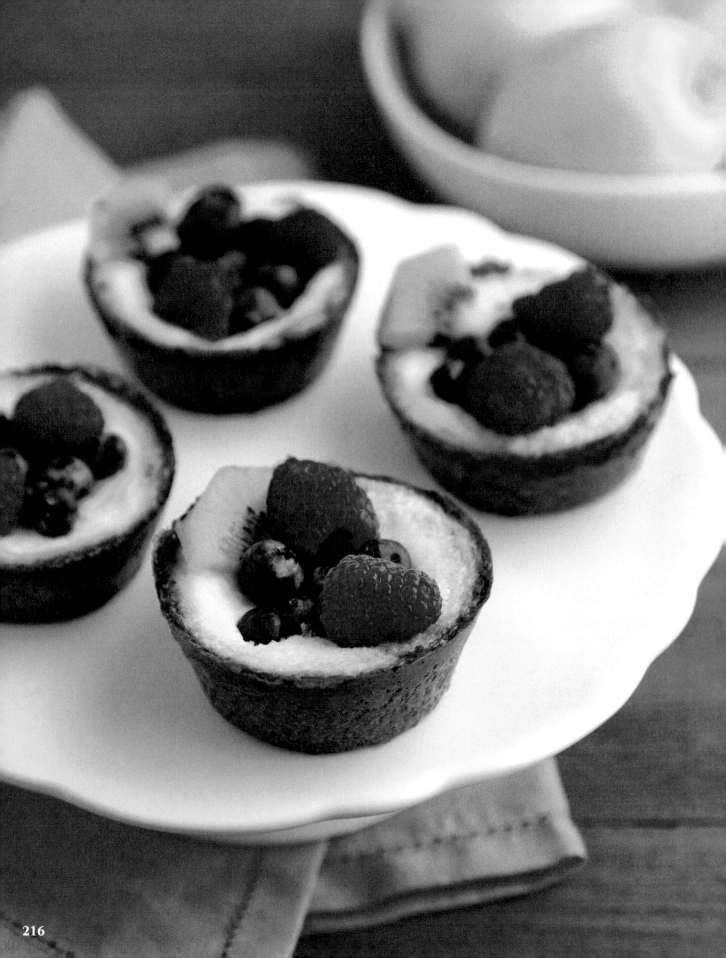

MINI FRUIT TARTS
WITH LEMON CUSTARD

After developing more than 100 low-carb desserts, these beautiful and delicious custard cups are actually the first time we've ever made a fruit tart. The photo really speaks for itself on this one, but I think you'd rather taste it than see it!

SHOPPING LIST

Nonstick cooking spray
½ cup fresh berries, to top (see tip)

CRUST

2 cups blanched almond flour
¼ cup sugar substitute
2 tablespoons unsalted butter, softened
1 large egg

FILLING

1¼ cups half-and-half
¾ cup sugar substitute
2 large eggs
2 large egg yolks
1 tablespoon lemon juice
Zest of 1 lemon

HELPFUL TIPS

We like to use a combination of fresh berries, and a small slice of kiwi to top these.

1 PLACE oven rack in the center position and preheat to 350°F. Spray a 12-cup muffin pan with nonstick cooking spray.

2 PLACE all Crust ingredients in a food processor, and pulse until a dough is formed.

3 USE your fingers to roll the dough into 12 equal balls. Place a ball of dough in each of the muffin cups, cover with plastic wrap, and press down to spread evenly across the bottom of each cup. Discard plastic wrap.

4 BAKE crust for 10–12 minutes, until lightly browned. Let cool as you prepare the Filling.

5 ADD Filling ingredients to a blender and blend 30 seconds, until smooth.

6 TOP the cooked crust in each muffin cup with an equal amount of the Filling.

7 BAKE for 25–30 minutes, or until the centers are mostly set. Let cool on a wire rack for 30 minutes.

8 TOP with an equal amount of the fresh berries, cover, and refrigerate for at least 1 hour before serving.

DESSERTS

WHAT MAKES IT QUICK & EASY: We skipped the stovetop! Traditionally, custard has to be carefully made on the stove and can lead to scrambled eggs without constant mixing.

Calories: 195 • Fat: 16g • Protein: 7g • Total Carbs: 8g − Fiber: 2g = **Net Carbs: 6g**

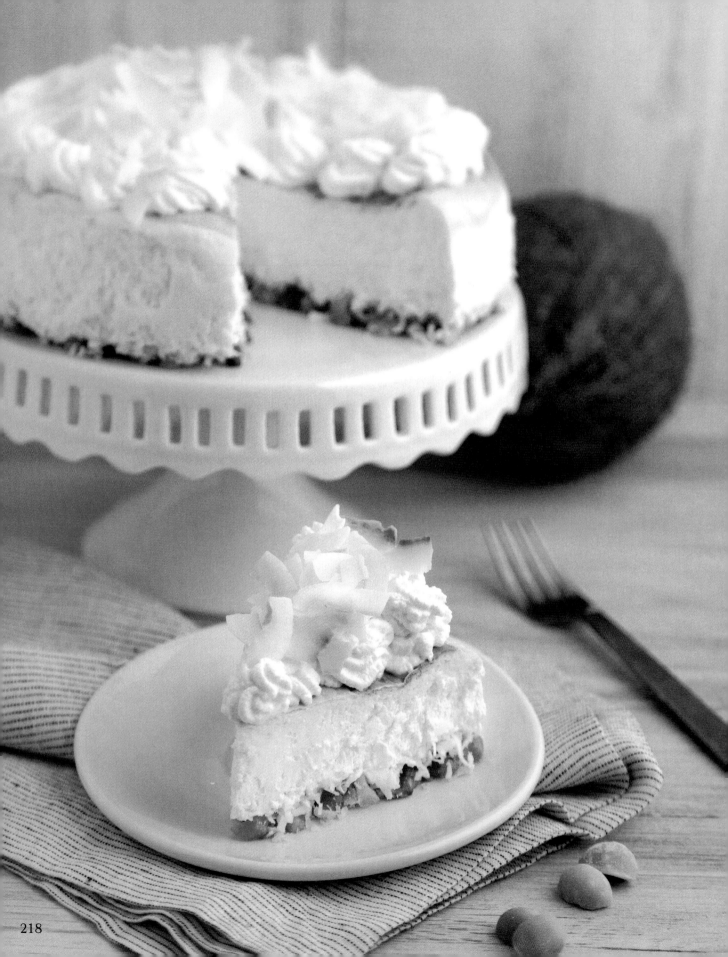

COCONUT CHEESECAKE
WITH MACADAMIA NUT CRUST

It's a taste of the tropics with this beautiful cheesecake featuring a macadamia nut crust and 3 bursts of coconut: shredded coconut, coconut milk, and coconut extract.

SHOPPING LIST

Nonstick cooking spray

1 cup shredded unsweetened coconut

¾ cup chopped macadamia nuts

24 ounces cream cheese, softened

1 cup sugar substitute

⅔ cup unsweetened coconut milk (not reduced-fat)

1 teaspoon coconut extract

1 teaspoon vanilla extract

3 large eggs

HELPFUL TIPS

We've had springform pans let water from the water bath seep into the pan, so we like to wrap the sides and bottom of the pan with aluminum foil, just in case.

1 PLACE oven rack in the center position and preheat to 350°F. Spray an 8-inch springform pan with nonstick cooking spray.

2 MAKE a water bath by pouring 1 inch of hot water into a shallow roasting pan. Place the water bath onto the center oven rack to preheat.

3 SPRINKLE the unsweetened coconut and macadamia nuts evenly over the bottom of the greased springform pan.

4 PLACE the cream cheese, sugar substitute, coconut milk, coconut extract, and vanilla extract in an electric mixer, and mix on medium speed, until combined.

5 ADD the eggs to the mixer, and continue mixing on medium, just until all is blended into a smooth filling.

6 SPREAD the filling over the coconut and nuts in the prepared springform pan.

7 PLACE pan in preheated water bath and bake for 1 hour 15 minutes, or until the top is light brown and the cake is pulling away from the sides of the pan.

8 COOL on a wire rack for 1 hour, then refrigerate at least 6 hours before slicing to serve.

DESSERTS

WHAT MAKES IT QUICK & EASY: After much testing, I was able to cut the baking time down by 30 minutes compared to cheesecakes in my previous books.

Calories: 355 · Fat: 34g · Protein: 7.5g · Total Carbs: 7.5g – Fiber: 3g = **Net Carbs: 4.5g**

RECIPE INDEX

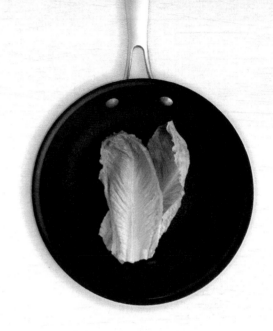

BREAKFAST

LUNCH

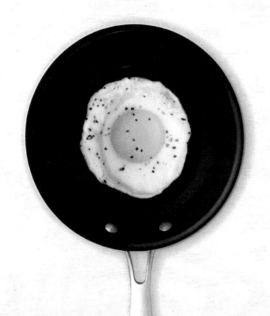

APPETIZERS & SNACKS

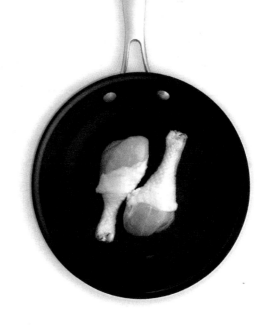

POULTRY

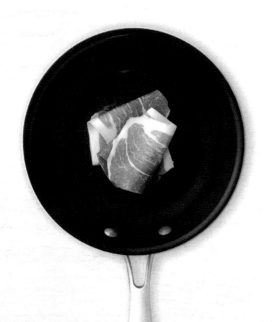

RECIPE INDEX
CONTINUED

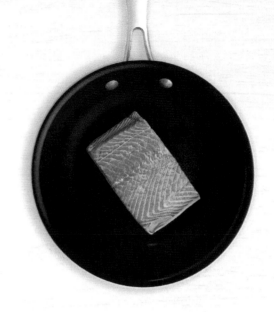

MEATS

SEAFOOD

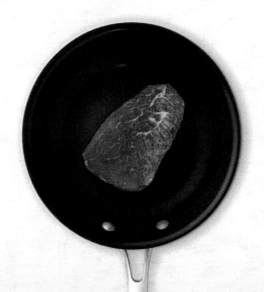

SIDE DISHES

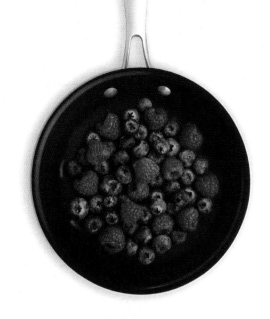

DESSERTS

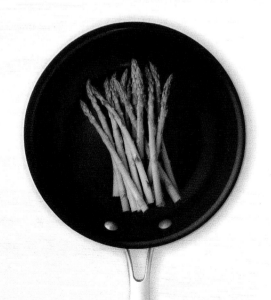

ABOUT THE AUTHOR

George Stella has been a professional chef for over 30 years. He has appeared on numerous television and news shows, including two seasons of his own show, *Low Carb and Lovin' It*, on the Food Network. Most recently he appeared on *The Dr. Oz Show* for a profile on the comfort foods the Stella family reinvented using unique and low-carb alternatives to white flour and sugar.

Connecticut born, George has spent more than half of his life in Florida, where he lives today, with his wife Rachel. This is his eighth cookbook.

To keep up to date on George, please visit:

www.StellaStyle.com

ABOUT THE PHOTOGRAPHY

The food photographs and design of this book were done by **Christian and Elise Stella**, George's son and daughter-in-law. They have worked previously on the design and photography of twenty cookbooks for various authors. They are frequent collaborators with Bob Warden and designed, photographed, and co-authored his bestselling cookbook *Great Food Fast*.

All food in the photographs was purchased at an ordinary grocery store or grown in Rachel's garden. Dishes were prepared to the recipe's directions. No artificial food styling techniques were used to "enhance" the food's appearance.